Management of
PHACO COMPLICATIONS
Newer Techniques

System requirement:
- Operating System—Windows XP or above.
- Web Browser—Internet Explorer 8 or above, Google Chrome, Mozilla Firefox.
- Essential plugins—Java and Flash Player.
    - Facing problems in viewing content—it may be your system does not have Java enabled.
    - If videos do not show up—it may be the system requires Flash Player or need to manage Flash setting. To learn more about Flash setting click on the link in the help section.
    - You can test Java and Flash by using the links from the help section of the **CD/DVD**.

Accompanying DVD-ROMS is playable only in Computer and not in DVD player.
CD/DVD has autorun function—it may take few seconds to load on your computer. If it does not work for you, then follow the steps below to access the contents manually:
- Click on my computer.
- Select the **CD/DVD** drive and click open/explore—this will show list of files in the **CD/DVD**.
- Find and double click file—"launch.html".

For more information about troubleshoot of autorun click on:
http://support.microsoft.com/kb/330135

DVD Contents

DVD 1
1. Descemet's detachment
2. Descemet's membrane endothelial keratoplasty (DMEK) with glued intraocular lens (IOL)
3. Dropped nucleus
4. Glued intraocular lens (IOL) scaffolding
5. Handshake technique for glued intraocular lens (IOL)

DVD 2
1. *Lessons learned:* Complications of glued intraocular lens (IOL)
2. Longest day 1
3. Pre-Descemet's endothelial keratoplasty (PDEK) with glued intraocular lens (IOL)
4. Intraocular lens (IOL) scaffold technique
5. Longest day 2
6. Three times haptic breaking to glued intraocular lens (IOL) with two months postoperative

Management of
PHACO COMPLICATIONS
Newer Techniques

Editor-in-Chief

Amar Agarwal MS FRCS FRCOphth
Chairman and Managing Director
Dr Agarwal's Group of Eye Hospitals and Eye Research Center
Chennai, Tamil Nadu, India

Co-Editor

Priya Narang MS
Medical Director
Narang Eye Care and Laser Center
Ahmedabad, Gujarat, India

Foreword

Arthur Cummings

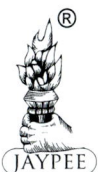

JAYPEE BROTHERS MEDICAL PUBLISHERS (P) LTD
New Delhi • London • Philadelphia • Panama

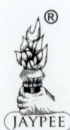

Jaypee Brothers Medical Publishers (P) Ltd.

Headquarters
Jaypee Brothers Medical Publishers (P) Ltd.
4838/24, Ansari Road, Daryaganj
New Delhi 110 002, India
Phone: +91-11-43574357
Fax: +91-11-43574314
Email: jaypee@jaypeebrothers.com

Overseas Offices

J.P. Medical Ltd.
83, Victoria Street, London
SW1H 0HW (UK)
Phone: +44-2031708910
Fax: +02-03-0086180
Email: info@jpmedpub.com

Jaypee-Highlights Medical Publishers Inc.
City of Knowledge, Bld. 237, Clayton
Panama City, Panama
Phone: +1 507-301-0496
Fax: +1 507-301-0499
Email: cservice@jphmedical.com

Jaypee Medical Inc.
The Bourse
111, South Independence Mall East
Suite 835, Philadelphia, PA 19106, USA
Phone: +1 267-519-9789
Email: jpmed.us@gmail.com

Jaypee Brothers Medical Publishers (P) Ltd.
17/1-B, Babar Road, Block-B, Shaymali
Mohammadpur, Dhaka-1207
Bangladesh
Mobile: +08801912003485
Email: jaypeedhaka@gmail.com

Jaypee Brothers Medical Publishers (P) Ltd.
Bhotahity, Kathmandu, Nepal
Phone: +977-9741283608
Email: kathmandu@jaypeebrothers.com

Website: www.jaypeebrothers.com
Website: www.jaypeedigital.com

© 2014, Jaypee Brothers Medical Publishers

The views and opinions expressed in this book are solely those of the original contributor(s)/author(s) and do not necessarily represent those of editor(s) of the book.

All rights reserved. No part of this publication and DVD-ROMs may be reproduced, stored or transmitted in any form or by any means, electronic, mechanical, photocopying, recording or otherwise, without the prior permission in writing of the publishers.

All brand names and product names used in this book are trade names, service marks, trademarks or registered trademarks of their respective owners. The publisher is not associated with any product or vendor mentioned in this book.

Medical knowledge and practice change constantly. This book is designed to provide accurate, authoritative information about the subject matter in question. However, readers are advised to check the most current information available on procedures included and check information from the manufacturer of each product to be administered, to verify the recommended dose, formula, method and duration of administration, adverse effects and contraindications. It is the responsibility of the practitioner to take all appropriate safety precautions. Neither the publisher nor the author(s)/editor(s) assume any liability for any injury and/or damage to persons or property arising from or related to use of material in this book.

This book is sold on the understanding that the publisher is not engaged in providing professional medical services. If such advice or services are required, the services of a competent medical professional should be sought.

Every effort has been made where necessary to contact holders of copyright to obtain permission to reproduce copyright material. If any have been inadvertently overlooked, the publisher will be pleased to make the necessary arrangements at the first opportunity.

Inquiries for bulk sales may be solicited at: jaypee@jaypeebrothers.com

Management of PHACO Complications: Newer Techniques

First Edition: **2014**

ISBN: 978-93-5152-151-8

Printed at : Samrat Offset Pvt Ltd.

Dedicated to

Donald Tan

A great surgeon and human being

Contributors

Amar Agarwal MS FRCS FRCOphth
Chairman and Managing Director
Dr Agarwal's Group of Eye Hospitals and
Eye Research Center
Chennai, Tamil Nadu, India

Ashvin Agarwal MS
Director
Dr Agarwal's Group of Eye Hospitals and
Eye Research Center
Chennai, Tamil Nadu, India

Brian Little MD FRCS FRCOphth
Consultant
Moorfield's Eye Hospital
London, UK

Dhivya Ashok Kumar MD
Consultant
Dr Agarwal's Group of Eye Hospitals and
Eye Research Center
Chennai, Tamil Nadu, India

George Beiko BM BCh FRCS(C)
Assistant Professor of Ophthalmology
McMaster University, St Catharines
Ontario, Canada

Nicole R Fram MD
Advanced Vision Care
Los Angeles
California, USA

Priya Narang MS
Medical Director
Narang Eye Care and Laser Center
Ahmedabad, Gujarat, India

Roger Steinert MD
Director
The Gavin Herbert Eye Institute
Department of Ophthalmology
University of California
Irvine, California, USA

Samuel Masket MD
Advanced Vision Care
David Geffen School of Medicine
Ucla, Jules Stein Eye Institute
Los Angeles, California, USA

Toshihiko Ohta MD PhD
Assistant Professor
Department of Ophthalmology
Juntendo University Shizuoka Hospital
Shizuoka, Japan

Foreword

When Dr Amar Agarwal invited me to write the foreword for *Management of PHACO Complications: Newer Techniques*, my first thought was "Is there anything more one can say about this prolific ophthalmologist that has not already been said?" On reflection, however, I do not know of anyone that is more productive in our field and what's more, who has opinions that are all based on their own work and experience. Having said 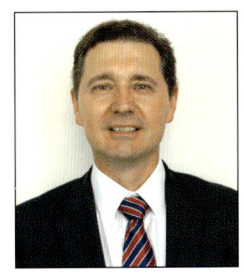 that, he is the first to acknowledge even the smallest contribution that any colleague has made to improve any of his surgical skills. With that in mind, what could have been a daunting task instead becomes pretty straight forward and my absolute pleasure and honor.

Dr Agarwal has a curriculum vitae as long as I have seen and is widely published, has authored or edited 56 previous ophthalmic texts and has presented hundreds of lectures all over the globe. His videos are incredibly well filmed, edited to show everything during the surgical procedure, whether good, great or not so good and hence land up becoming teaching tools of significant value. He has contributed with new surgical instruments, surgical devices and novel techniques, and he and his hospital group have discovered or developed at least 30 new inventions that have led to ophthalmic surgeons worldwide being better equipped to deal with cataract surgery and beyond. As though, this is not enough, he serves on numerous committees and boards and in many, in a chairing role. At the time this book is being published, Dr Agarwal is the current International Society of Refractive Surgery (ISRS) President. All of the aforementioned are incredibly impressive but is still not, for me at least, the most impressive aspect of Dr Agarwal's work. The reader may notice that Dr Agarwal, even though, he may consult for industry, does not push any one product or company but is rather behoved to nothing but the absolute truth. Whenever he tells you something, teaches you a new technique, writes a new article or book, it is only the facts that become apparent. There are no other motives. An extremely affable man, Dr Agarwal's sense of humor, genuine love for his profession, patients and colleagues allows him to enjoy the admiration and respect of the international ophthalmic community. Anterior segment surgery would not be the same today were, it not for his contributions; such is the extent of his impact on our field. It is to our benefit that he has chosen to share his vast repertoire of skills by means of writing, presenting lectures and showing surgical videos, and many thousands of ophthalmic surgeons worldwide are grateful for this.

Dr Agarwal has not only edited the book, but also together with Dr Priya Narang, has basically written the book. There are only a few chapters not written by one or both of these two editors in the entire book. Dr Narang is an accomplished surgeon, author, researcher and contributor to ophthalmology in her own right, and together with Dr Agarwal, they have produced a comprehensive work that will certainly provide the cataract surgeon with more options when complications are encountered. There are some contributions from invited international experts in their respective fields of cataract surgery that simply rounds off a superb work on the vast topic of phaco surgery and new techniques of managing complications. As with almost all of his preceding works, this one is destined to become another best seller for this remarkable colleague. I know that if you gain only 10 percent of the intended transfer of knowledge contained in Dr Agarwal's latest book, you will become a more competent cataract surgeon.

Arthur Cummings MD FRCS Ed
Medical Director
Wellington Eye Clinic
Dublin, Ireland

Preface

With the technologies vying for a place in a surgeon's practice while accentuating the surgical precision and results; the scope for complications although minimized, still exists. Ophthalmologists often go through sleepless nights in pursuit of choosing a correct technique to handle their complications and optimizing the visual output. The aim of the book is to provide tangible evidence on the changes in the procedures for cataract care and surgical technique.

The book is a result of commitment to innovation and excellence in ophthalmology. It explains in detail, the different surgical methods and innovations in tackling complications of cataract surgery aimed at achieving ultimate individualization of management of cases. Further, it enhances a deeper understanding of the fundamental surgical principles, as well as the minute surgical technical details of a complicated scenario. The book entails:

- Informative figures and illustrations
- Highlights the latest surgical techniques for managing complications in cataract surgery
- Customizes the surgical technique for each patient
- DVDs of surgical techniques to facilitate proper understanding of the technique.

We would like to extend our special thanks to all members of M/s Jaypee Brothers Medical Publishers (P) Ltd, New Delhi, India, for their intense effort for publication and promotion of the book.

Amar Agarwal
Priya Narang

Acknowledgment

Nothing in this world moves without HIM and so the book is only written by HIM.

Contents

Section I: Interventions in Posterior Capsular Rupture

1. **Gas Forced Infusion: Controlling the Surge** 3
   Amar Agarwal
   History *3*
   Introduction *4*
   Technique *5*
   Method *5*

2. **Posterior Capsular Rupture** 10
   Dhivya Ashok Kumar, Amar Agarwal
   Common Risk Factors for Posterior Capsular Rupture *10*
   Steps for Management of Posterior Capsular Rupture *12*
   Sequelae after Posterior Capsular Rupture *16*

3. **Pars Plicata Anterior Vitrectomy: A Redefined Approach** 23
   Priya Narang, Amar Agarwal
   Anatomic Considerations *23*
   Surgical Technique *25*
   Precautions *27*

4. **Sleeveless Phacotip Assisted Levitation of Dropped Nucleus** 30
   Priya Narang, Amar Agarwal
   Surgical Technique *31*

5. **Sleeveless Extrusion Cannula for Levitation of Dropped Intraocular Lens** 39
   Ashvin Agarwal, Priya Narang, Amar Agarwal
   Surgical Technique *39*

Section II: Glued Intraocular Lens and Intraocular Lens Scaffold

6. Glued Intrascleral Haptic Fixation of Intraocular Lens (Glued IOL) — 47
Ashvin Agarwal, Amar Agarwal
White To White Measurement *47*
Surgical Technique *47*

7. Handshake Technique for Glued IOL — 65
Priya Narang, Amar Agarwal
Leading Haptic Externalization *65*
Trailing Haptic Externalization *65*
Scharioth Tuck and Glue *67*
Injector *67*
Handshake Technique for Foldable Glued IOL *67*

8. Modifications in the Glued Intraocular Lens Technique — 72
Priya Narang, George Beiko, Toshihiko Ohta, Amar Agarwal
No-Assistant Technique *72*
Surgical Technique *74*
Beiko and Steinert's Modification *77*
Toshihiko Ohta's Y-Fixation Technique *79*
Problems with the Glued Intraocular Lens Technique and their Solutions *84*

9. Intraocular Lens Scaffold — 87
Priya Narang, Amar Agarwal
Surgical Technique *87*

10. Glued Intraocular Lens Scaffold — 92
Priya Narang, Amar Agarwal
Concept and Indications *92*
Surgical Technique *92*
Difficulties *101*

Section III: Miscellaneous

11. **Intraocular Lens Scaffold for Intraocular Lens Exchange** 105
    Roger Steinert, Brian Little, Priya Narang, Amar Agarwal
    Surgical Technique *106*

12. **Pre-Descemet's Endothelial Keratoplasty** 110
    Harminder Dua, Priya Narang, Amar Agarwal
    Surgical Technique *110*

13. **Negative Dysphotopsia** 115
    Samuel Masket, Nicole R Fram
    Negative Dysphotopsia *115*
    Positive Dysphotopsia *119*

Index 121

SECTION

I

Interventions in Posterior Capsular Rupture

CHAPTER 1

Gas Forced Infusion: Controlling the Surge

Amar Agarwal

HISTORY

The main problem encountered in bimanual phaco/phakonit was the destabilization of the anterior chamber during surgery. This was solved by us to a certain extent by using an 18-gauge irrigating chopper. Dr Sunita Agarwal suggested the use of an antichamber collapser, which injects air into the infusion bottle (Fig. 1.1). This pushes more fluid into the eye through the irrigating chopper and also prevents surge.[1-11] Thus, we were able to use a 20 gauge or 21 gauge irrigating chopper as well as solve the problem of destabilization of the anterior

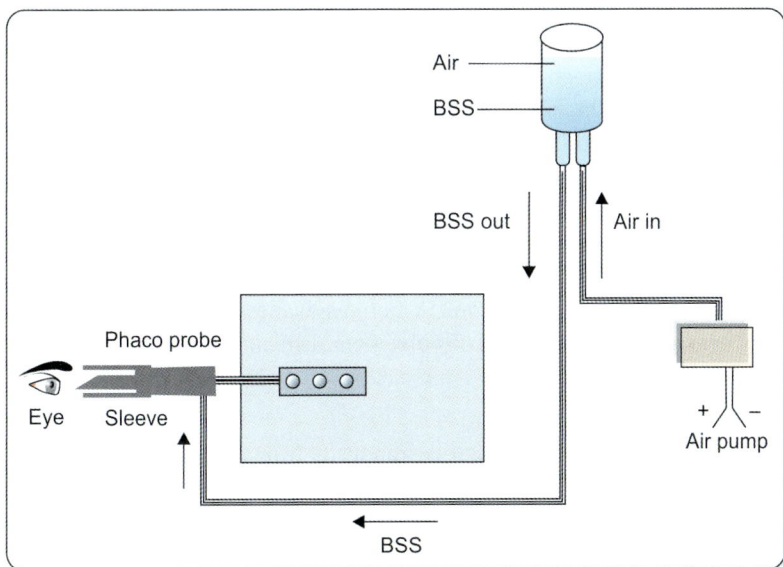

Fig. 1.1 Diagrammatic representation of the connection of the air pump to the infusion bottle
Abbreviation: BSS—Balanced salt solution

chamber during surgery. Now with microphakonit and gas forced infusion we are able to remove cataracts with a 0.7 mm irrigating chopper (22 gauge). Subsequently we used this system in all our co-axial phaco cases including microincisional co-axial phaco to prevent complications like posterior capsular ruptures and corneal damage.

INTRODUCTION

Since the introduction of phacoemulsification by Kelman,[1] it has been undergoing revolutionary changes in an attempt to perfect the techniques of extracapsular cataract extraction surgery. Although advantageous in many aspects, this technique is not without its attending complications. A well-maintained anterior chamber without intraocular fluctuations is one of the prerequisites for safe phacoemulsification and phakonit.[2]

When an occluded fragment is held by high vacuum and then abruptly aspirated, fluid rushes into the phaco tip to equilibrate the built up vacuum in the aspiration line, causing surge.[3] This leads to shallowing or collapse of the anterior chamber. Different machines employ a variety of methods to combat surge. These include usage of noncompliant tubing,[4] small bore aspiration line tubing,[4] microflow tips,[4] aspiration bypass systems,[4] dual linear foot pedal control[4] and incorporation of sophisticated microprocessors[4] to sense the anterior chamber pressure fluctuations.

The surgeon dependent variables to counteract surge include good wound construction with minimal leakage,[5] and selection of appropriate machine parameters depending on the stage of the surgery.[5] An anterior chamber maintainer has also been described in literature to prevent surge, but an extra side port makes it an inconvenient procedure.

We started a simple and effective method to prevent anterior chamber collapse during phacoemulsification and phakonit in 1999 by increasing the velocity of the fluid inflow into the anterior chamber. This is achieved by an automated air pump which pumps atmospheric air through an air filter into the infusion bottle thereby preventing surge. We stumbled upon this idea when we were operating cases with phakonit[7] where we wanted more fluid entering the eye, but even now we use it in all our phacoemulsification cases.[8]

Air Pump

An automated air pump is used to push air into the infusion bottle thus increasing the pressure with which the fluid flows into the eye. This increases the steady-state pressure of the eye making the anterior chamber deep and well-maintained during the entire procedure. It makes phakonit and phacoemulsification a relatively safe procedure by reducing surge even at high vacuum levels.

TECHNIQUE

A locally manufactured automated device, used in fish tanks (aquariums) to supply oxygen, is utilized to forcefully pump air into the irrigation bottle. This pump is available in aquarium shops and has an electromagnetic motor which moves a lever attached to a collapsible rubber cap. There is an inlet with a valve, which sucks in atmospheric air as the cap expands. On collapsing, the valve closes and the air is pushed into an intravenous (IV) line connected to the infusion bottle (Fig. 1.1). The lever vibrates at a frequency of approximately 10 oscillations per second. The electromagnetic motor is weak enough to stop once the pressure in the closed system (i.e. the anterior chamber) reaches about 50 mm of Hg. The rubber cap ceases to expand at this pressure level. A millipore air filter is used between the air pump and the infusion bottle so that the air pumped into the bottle is clean of the particulate matter.

METHOD

- First of all, the balanced salt solution (BSS) bottle is taken and put on the IV stand.
- Now we take an air pump. This air pump is the kind which is used in fish tanks (aquariums) to infuse oxygen to the fishes. The air pump is plugged on to the electrical connection.
- An IV set now connects the air pump to the infusion bottle. The tubing passes from the air pump and the end of the tubing is passed into one of the infusion bottles.
- When the air pump is switched on, it pumps air into the infusion bottle. This air goes to the top of the bottle and because of the pressure; it pumps the fluid down with greater force. With this, the fluid now flows from the infusion bottle to reach the phaco handpiece or irrigating chopper. The amount of fluid now coming out of the handpiece is much more than what would normally come out and with more force.
- A millipore air filter is connected between the air pump and the infusion bottle so that the air which is being pumped into the bottle is sterile.
- This extra amount of fluid coming out compensates for the surge which would otherwise occur.

Continuous Infusion

Before we enter the eye, we fill the eye with viscoelastic. Then once the tip of the phaco handpiece in phaco or irrigating chopper in phakonit is inside the anterior chamber we shift to continuous irrigation. This is very helpful especially for surgeons who are in the learning curve of phacoemulsification or phakonit. This way, the surgeon never comes to position zero and the anterior chamber never collapses. Even for excellent surgeons this helps a lot.

Advantages

- With the air pump, the posterior capsule is pushed back and there is a deep anterior chamber.
- The phenomenon of surge is neutralized and this in turn prevents posterior capsular rupture.
- Striate keratitis postoperatively is reduced, as there is a deep anterior chamber.
- Hard cataracts can be operated quite comfortably, as striate keratitis does not occur postoperatively.
- The surgical time is shorter as one can emulsify the nuclear pieces much faster as surge does not occur.
- One can easily operate cases with the phakonit technique as quite a lot of fluid now passes into the eye. Thus, the cataract can be removed through a smaller opening.
- It is quite comfortable to do cases under topical or no-anesthesia.

Topical or No-Anesthesia Cataract Surgery

During phacoemulsification under topical or no-anesthesia, the main problem encountered is that sometimes the pressure is high especially if the patient squeezes the eye. In such cases, the posterior capsule comes up anteriorly and one can produce a posterior capsular rupture. To solve this problem, surgeons tend to work more anteriorly, performing supracapsular phacoemulsification/phakonit. The disadvantage of this is that striate keratitis tends to occur.

With the air pump, this problem is solved totally as the posterior capsule is pushed back. In other words, there is a lot of space between the posterior capsule and the cornea, preventing striate keratitis and inadvertent posterior capsular rupture.

Internal Gas Forced Infusion

This was started by Arturo Pérez-Arteaga from Mexico. The anterior vented gas forced infusion system (AVGFI) of the Accurus surgical system is used.

This is a system incorporated in the Accurus machine that creates a positive infusion pressure inside the eye; it was designed by the Alcon engineers to control the intraocular pressure (IOP) during posterior segment surgery. It consist of an air pump and a regulator which are inside the machine; then the air is pushed inside the bottle of intraocular solution, and so the fluid is actively pushed inside the eye without raising or lowering the bottle. The control of the air pump is digitally integrated in the Accurus panel; it also can be controlled via the remote. Also the footswitch can be preset with the minimal and maximum of desired fluid inside the eye and go directly to this value with the simple touch of the footswitch. Arturo Pérez-Arteaga recommends to preset the infusion pump at 100 mm of Hg; it is enough strong irrigation force to perform a microincision phaco. This parameter is preset in the panel and also as the minimal irrigation force in the footswitch; then he recommends to preset the maximum irrigation force at 130

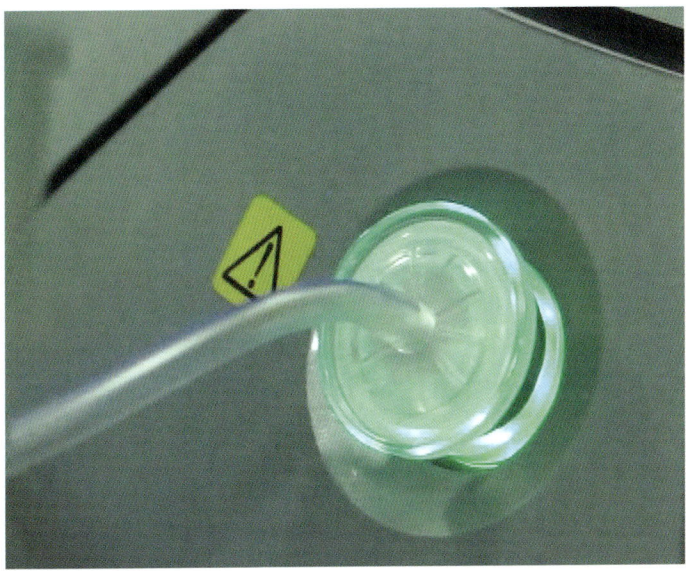

Fig. 1.2 Millipore filter to connect the air pump to the tubing. Air pump in the Stellaris (Bausch and Lomb) machine

to 140 mm of Hg in the foot pedal, so if a surge exist during the procedure the surgeon can increase the irrigation force by the simple touch of the footswitch to the right. With the AVGFI the surgeon has the capability to increase even more these values. A millipore filter is used again between the tubing and the air pump (Fig. 1.2).

Stellaris Pressurized Infusion System

Bausch and Lomb have installed air pump in their Stellaris machine in 2009. The advantage of this is that one has an internal gas forced infusion now as the air pump which was an external gas forced infusion system is now inside the machine (Fig. 1.3). Another advantage is there is a monitor in the panel of the machine and one can lower or raise the pressure of the air pump.

Centurion active fluidics by Alcon: Active fluidics allows the surgeon to set and maintain the appropriate intraocular pressure (IOP). The system has dual pressure laser sensors to detect irrigation pressure and aspiration vacuum to maintain the target IOP. It also has rotatory valves and dual segment pump designed for smooth flow.

DISCUSSION

Surge is defined as the volume of the fluid forced out of the eye into the aspiration line at the instant of occlusion break. When the phacoemulsification handpiece tip is occluded, flow is interrupted and vacuum builds up to its preset values.

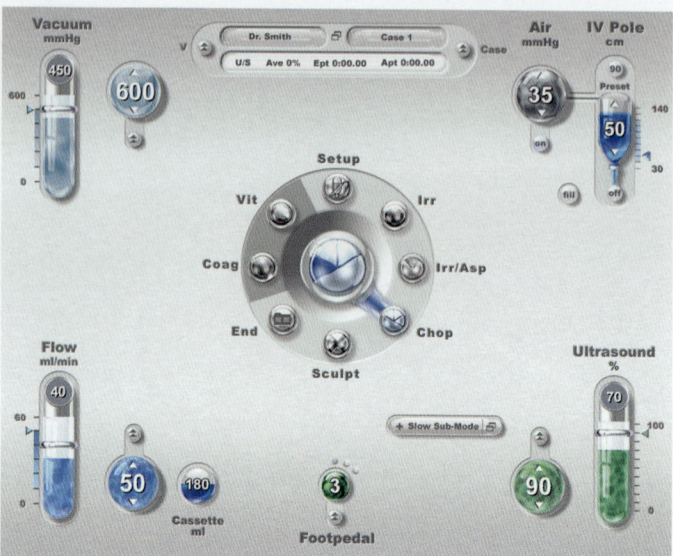

Fig. 1.3 Stellaris (Bausch and Lomb) pressurized infusion system. Note in the upper right corner IV pole height in cm and next to it shows the air pump (gas forced infusion pressure) in mm of Hg

Additionally, the aspiration tubing may collapse in the presence of high vacuum levels. Emulsification of the occluding fragment clears the block and the fluid rushes into the aspiration line to neutralize the pressure difference created between the positive pressure in the anterior chamber and the negative pressure in the aspiration tubing. In addition, if the aspiration line tubing is not reinforced to prevent collapse (tubing compliance), the tubing, constricted during occlusion, then expands on occlusion break. These factors cause a rush of fluid from the anterior chamber into the phaco probe. The fluid in the anterior chamber is not replaced rapidly enough to prevent shallowing of the anterior chamber.

The maintenance of intraocular pressure (steady-state IOP)[2] during the entire procedure depends on the equilibrium between the fluid inflow and outflow. The steady state pressure level is the mean pressure equilibrium between inflow and outflow volumes. In most phacoemulsification machines, fluid inflow is provided by gravitational flow of the fluid from the balanced salt solution (BSS) bottle through the tubing to the anterior chamber. This is determined by the bottle height relative to the patient's eye, the diameter of the tubing and most importantly by the outflow of fluid from the eye through the aspiration tube and leakage from the wounds.[2]

The inflow volume can be increased by either increasing the bottle height or by enlarging the diameter of the inflow tube. The intraocular pressure increases by 10 mm Hg for every 15 centimeters increase in bottle height above the eye.[5]

High steady-state IOPs increase phaco safety by raising the mean IOP level up and away from zero, i.e. by delaying surge related anterior chamber collapse.[2]

Air pump increases the amount of fluid inflow thus making the steady-state IOP high. This deepens the anterior chamber, increasing the surgical space available for maneuvering and thus prevents complications like posterior capsular tears and corneal endothelial damage. The phenomenon of surge is neutralized by rapid inflow of fluid at the time of occlusion break. The recovery to steady-state IOP is so prompt that no surge occurs and this enables the surgeon to remain in foot position 3 through the occlusion break. High vacuum phacoemulsification/ phakonit can be safely performed in hard brown cataracts using an air pump. Phacoemulsification or phakonit under topical or no-anesthesia[6, 7] can be safely done neutralizing the positive vitreous pressure occurring due to squeezing of the eyelids.

SUMMARY

The air pump is a new device, which helps to prevent surge. This prevents posterior capsular rupture, helps deepen the anterior chamber and makes phacoemulsification and phakonit a safe procedure even in hard cataracts.

REFERENCES

1. Kelman CD. Phacoemulsification and aspiration; a new technique of cataract removal; a preliminary report. Am J Ophthalmol. 1967;64:23-5.
2. Wilbrandt RH. Comparative analysis of the fluidics of the AMO Prestige, Alcon Legacy, and Storz Premiere phacoemulsification systems. J Cataract Refract Surg. 1997;23:766-80.
3. Seibel SB. Phacodynamics. Thorofare, NJ, Slack Inc. 1995;54.
4. Fishkind WJ. The Phaco Machine: How and why it acts and reacts? In: Agarwal's four volume textbook of Ophthalmology. Jaypee Brothers Medical Publishers (P) Ltd. New Delhi. 2000. (In print).
5. Seibel SB. The fluidics and physics of phaco. In: Agarwal's et al. Phacoemulsification, Laser cataract surgery and foldable IOLs, 2nd edn. Jaypee Brothers Medical Publishers (P) Ltd. New Delhi. 2000. pp. 45-54.
6. Agarwal, et al. No-anesthesia cataract surgery with karate chop. In: Agarwal's Phacoemulsification, Laser cataract surgery and foldable IOLs, 2nd edn. Jaypee Brothers Medical Publishers (P) Ltd. New Delhi. 2000. pp. 217-26.
7. Agarwal, et al. Phakonit and laser phakonit. In: Agarwal's Phacoemulsification, Laser cataract surgery and foldable IOLs, 2nd edn. Jaypee Brothers Medical Publishers (P) Ltd. New Delhi. 2000. pp. 204-16.
8. Agarwal A. Agarwal S. Agarwal A. Antichamber collapser. J Cataract Refract Surg. 2002;28:1085.
9. Agarwal A, Agarwal S, Agarwal A. Phakonit: phacoemulsification through a 0.9 mm incision. J Cataract Refract Surg. 2001;27:1548-52.
10. Agarwal A, Trivedi RH, Jacob S, et al. Microphakonit: 700 micron cataract surgery. Clin ophthal. 2007;1(3):323-5.
11. Agarwal A, Kumar DA, Jacob S, Agarwal A. In vivo analysis of wound architecture in 700 micron microphakonit surgery. J Cataract Refract Surg. 2008;34(9):1554-60.

CHAPTER 2

Posterior Capsular Rupture

Dhivya Ashok Kumar, Amar Agarwal

INTRODUCTION

Any breach in the continuity of the posterior capsule is defined as a posterior capsule tear. Intrasurgical posterior capsule tears are the most common and can occur during any stage of cataract surgery.[1,2,3] The incidence of posterior capsule complications is related to the type of cataract and conditions of the eye, increases with the grade of difficulty of the case, and furthermore is influenced by the level of experience of the surgeon. Timely recognition and a planned management, depending upon the stage of surgery during which the posterior capsule tear has occurred, is required to ensure an optimal visual outcome.

COMMON RISK FACTORS FOR POSTERIOR CAPSULAR RUPTURE

The common risk factors for posterior capsular rupture (PCR) are as follows:
- Intraoperative factors causing variation in anterior chamber depth
- Type of cataract
- Extended rhexis.

Intraoperative Factors Causing Variation in Anterior Chamber Depth

Intraoperative shallow anterior chamber could be due to various reasons. It may be a tight lid speculum, tight drapes, or pull from the recollecting bag. In all the above cases, remove the precipitating factor (Remove the speculum pressure, remove the tight drapes and collecting bags). Variation in the amount of space in the anterior and posterior chambers may result from changes in the intraocular pressure (IOP) due to an alteration in the equilibrium between inflow and outflow of fluid. Diminished inflow may be secondary to insufficient bottle height, tube occlusion or compression, bottle emptying, too tight incisions compressing the irrigation sleeve, or the surgeon moving the phaco tip out of the incision, making the irrigation holes come out of the incision. Excessive outflow may be caused by too high vacuum/flow parameters, or too large incisions with leakage. Another cause is the postocclusion surge. Use of air pump or gas forced infusion solves most of these problems of intraoperative shallow anterior chamber.[1]

Type of Cataract

A higher incidence of posterior capsule tear with vitreous loss is associated with cataract with pseudoexfoliation, diabetes mellitus, and trauma. Missing the diagnosis in a posterior polar cataract (Fig. 2.1) can be catastrophic to the surgeon and the patient. It is frequently associated with a weakened or deficient posterior capsule. Posterior lenticonus, cataracts with persistent primary hyperplastic vitreous, cataracts following vitreoretinal surgery and morgagnian cataracts are some of the other types. In any intraoperative diagnosis of posterior polar cataract, avoid hydrodissection with BSS. Hydrodissection may cause hydraulic perforation at the weakened area of the capsule, hence only a careful controlled hydrodelineation is preferred. One can also make multiple pockets of viscoelastic injection around the nucleus. If a capsular tear does occur, a closed system should be maintained by injecting viscoelastic before withdrawing the phaco tip. This helps to tamponade the vitreous backwards where a capsular dehiscence is present.

Extended Rhexis

Extension of anterior capsule can occur as a complication in MICS also. During capsulorhexis, anterior capsular tears can cause posterior capsule tear by

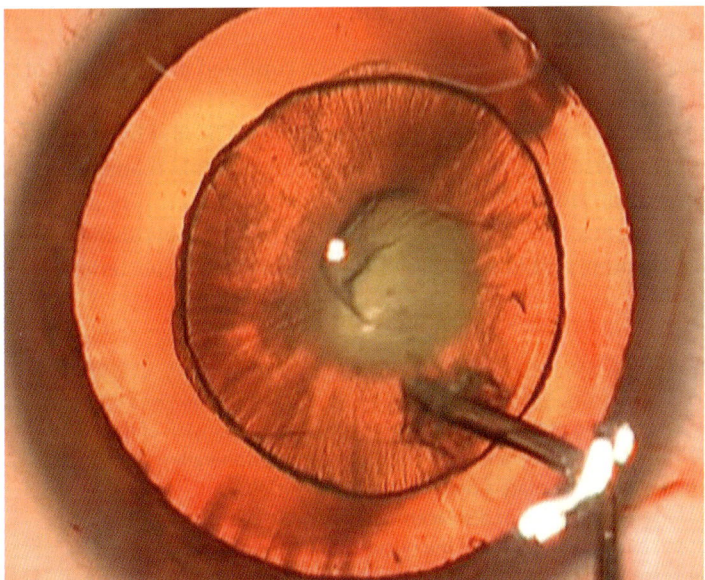

Fig. 2.1 Hydrodelineation is being performed in a posterior polar cataract

extending to the periphery. In a new method of managing this situation, a nick is made from the opposite side of the rhexis using a cystitome or vannas and the capsulorhexis is completed. The viscoelastic in the anterior chamber (AC) is then expressed out to make the globe hypotonous, following which a gentle hydrodissection is done at 90 degrees from the tear while pressing the posterior lip of the incision to prevent any rise in intraocular pressure (IOP). No attempt is made to press on the center of the nucleus to complete the fluid wave. The fluid is usually sufficient to prolapse one pole of the nucleus out of the capsular bag; else it is removed by embedding the phacoemulsification probe, making sure not to exert any downward pressure and then gently pulling the nucleus anteriorly. The whole nucleus is brought out into the AC and no nuclear division techniques are tried in the bag. The entire nucleus is prolapsed into the anterior chamber and emulsified.

STEPS FOR MANAGEMENT OF POSTERIOR CAPSULAR RUPTURE

Surgeon should be aware of the signs (Table 2.1) of posterior capsular tear. Posterior capsule tears can occur during any stage of phacoemulsification surgery. They occurred most frequently during the stage of nuclear emulsification, as reported by Mulhern et al [4] (49%) and Osher et al [5], and during irrigation–aspiration, as reported by Gimbel et al[6].

Three possible situations can happen in a posterior capsule rent namely[7]:
1. Posterior capsule tear with hyaloid face intact and nuclear material present.
2. Posterior capsule tear with hyaloid face ruptured without luxation of nuclear material into vitreous.
3. Posterior capsule tear with hyaloid face ruptured and luxation of nuclear material into vitreous.

Immediate precautions are to be taken not to do further hydrate the vitreous and not to increase the size of the PCR. The conventional management consists of prevention of mixture of cortical matter with vitreous, dry aspiration, and anterior vitrectomy, if required. In addition, during phacoemulsification low flow rate, high vacuum, and low ultrasound are advocated if a posterior capsule tear occurs.

TABLE 2.1 Signs of posterior capsular rupture (PCR)
- Sudden deepening of the chamber, with momentary expansion of the pupil
- Sudden, transitory appearance of a clear red reflex peripherally
- Apparent inability to rotate a previously mobile nucleus
- Excessive lateral mobility or displacement of the nucleus
- Excessive tipping of one pole of the nucleus
- Partial descent of the nucleus into the anterior vitreous space
- 'Pupil snap sign'—sudden marked pupil constriction after hydrodissection

Posterior Capsular Rupture

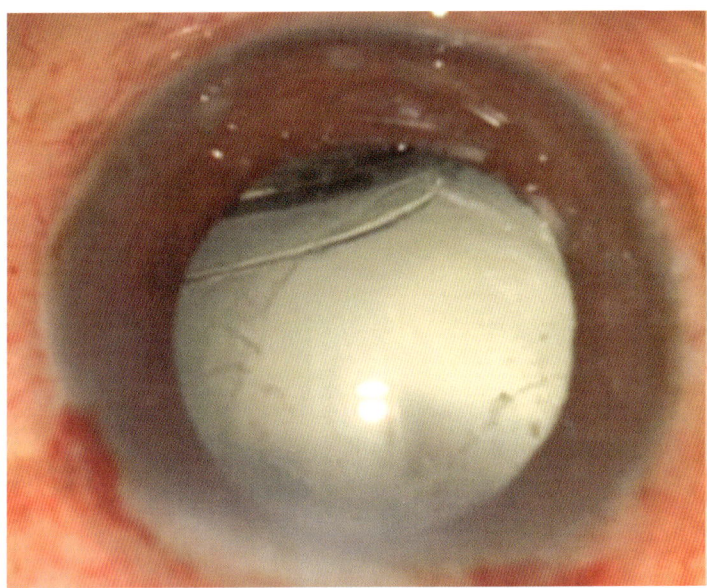

Fig. 2.2 Posterior capsular rupture. Note the IOL sinking into the vitreous cavity. The white reflex indicates nuclear fragments also in the vitreous cavity. This patient was managed by vitrectomy, SPAL technique (for removal of the nuclear fragments) and the IOL repositioned in the sulcus

Reduce the parameters: Lowering aspiration flow rate and decreasing the vacuum will control surge and will allow the bottle to be lowered, diminishing turbulence inside the eye. If the nucleus is soft, only a small residual amount remains, and there is no vitreous prolapse, the procedure may be continued. If vitreous is already present, special care must be taken for preventing additional vitreous prolapse into the anterior chamber or to the wound. Small residual nucleus or cortex can be emulsified by bringing it out of the capsular bag and can be emulsified in the anterior chamber with viscoelastic underneath the corneal endothelium. In case of a small PCR and minimal residual nucleus (Fig. 2.2), a dispersive viscoelastic is injected to plug the posterior capsule tear. Subsequently the nuclear material is moved into the anterior chamber with a spatula and emulsified. The recommended parameters are low bottle height (20–40 cm above the patient's head), low flow rate (10–15 cc/min), high vacuum (120–200 mm Hg) and low ultrasound (20–40%).

Dry cortical aspiration: If there is only a small amount or no vitreous prolapse in the presence of a small capsular rent, a dry cortical aspiration with 23 G cannula can be performed.

Viscoexpression: It is a method of removal of the residual nucleus by injecting viscoelastic underneath the nucleus to support it and the nucleus is expressed along with the viscoelastic.

Management of PHACO Complications: Newer Techniques

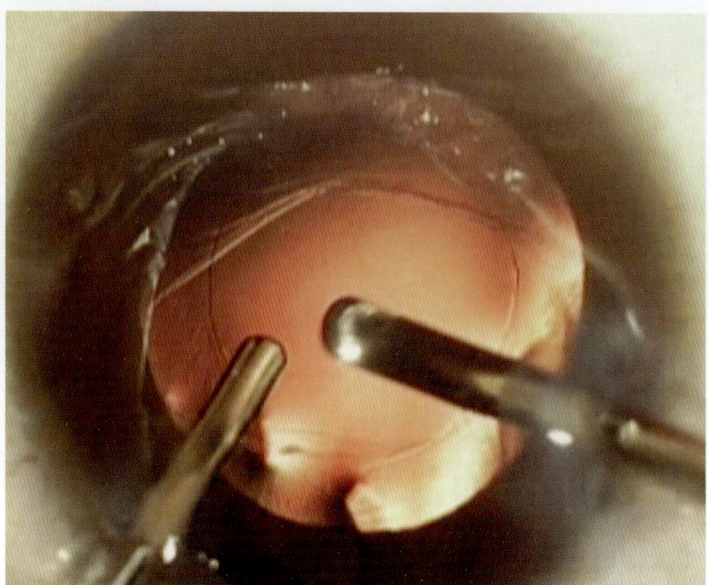

Fig. 2.3 Bimanual vitrectomy is being performed in a posterior capsular tear with vitreous prolapse

Conversion to ECCE: If there is sizeable amount of residual nucleus, it is advisable to convert to a large incision ECCE to minimize the possibility of a dropped nucleus.

Anterior bimanual vitrectomy: Bimanual vitrectomy (Fig. 2.3) is done in eyes with vitreous prolapse. Use 23 G irrigating cannula via side port after extending the side port incision. The irrigation bottle is positioned at the appropriate height to maintain the anterior chamber during vitrectomy. Vitrectomy should be performed with cutting rate (500–800 cuts per minute), an aspiration flow rate of 20 cc/min, and a vacuum of 150 to 200 mm Hg.

Anterior chamber cleared of vitreous: Vitrectomy is continued in the anterior chamber and the pupillary plane. A rod can be introduced into the anterior chamber to check the presence of any vitreous traction and the same should be released. Complete removal of the vitreous from the anterior chamber can be confirmed if you see a circular, mobile pupil (Figs 2.4A and B) and complete air bubble in the anterior chamber. The usage of the fiber of an endoilluminator, dimming the room lights and microscope lights, may be useful in cases of doubt, in order to identify vitreous strands. Another useful measure is the use of purified triamcinolone acetate suspension (Kenalog) to identify the vitreous described by Peyman [8]. Kenalog particles remain trapped on and within the vitreous gel, making it clearly visible.[9]

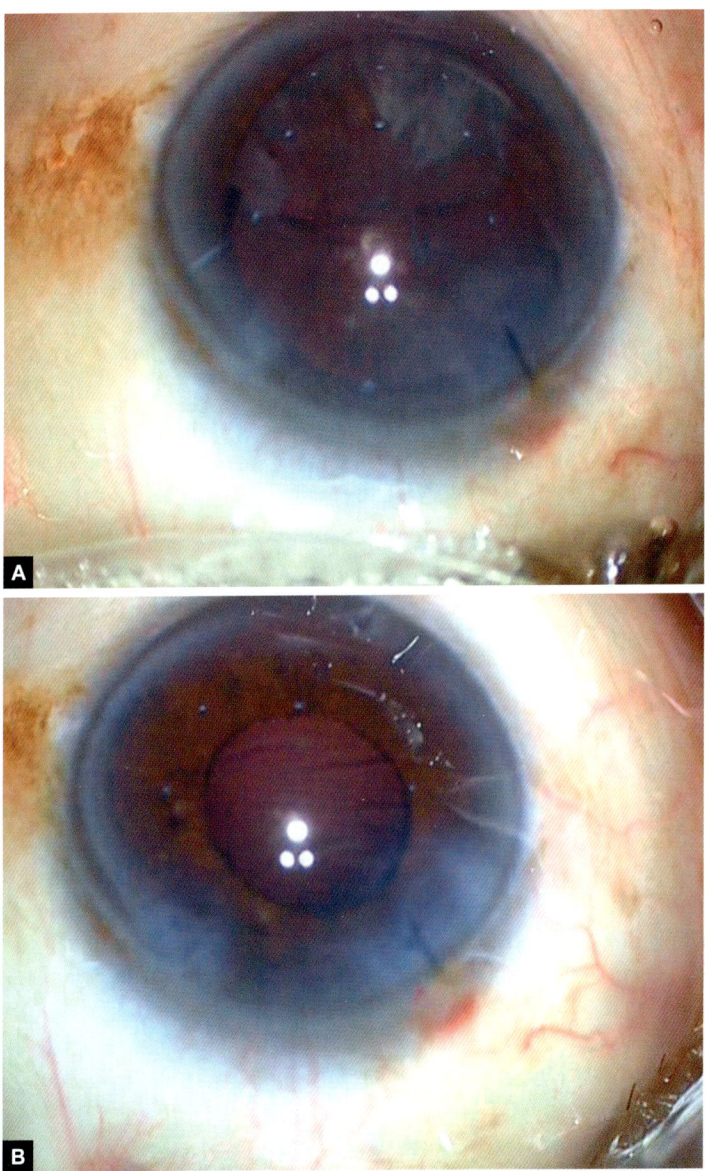

Figs 2.4A and B Clinical photograph showing the change in the anterior chamber after complete removal of the vitreous from the anterior chamber. (A) Before vitrectomy; (B) After vitrectomy

Suture the wound: In cases with vitreous loss with PCR, it is recommended to suture the corneal wound as a prophylaxis to prevent infection. Remove any residual vitreous in the incision site in the main and side port with vitrector or manually with vannas scissors. If necessary insert a rod via the side port, and pass it over the surface of the iris, to release them.

> **TABLE 2.2** Intraocular lens implantation in posterior capsular rupture
> - Insertion and rotation of IOL should always be away from the area of capsule tear
> - The long axis of the IOL should cross the meridian of the posterior capsule tear
> - Eyes with (< 6 mm) PCR with no vitreous loss, IOL can be placed in the capsular bag
> - In the presence of a posterior capsule tear (>6 mm) with adequate anterior capsule rim, an IOL can be placed in the sulcus
> - In deficient capsules, glued IOL is a promising technique without complications of sutured scleral fixated or anterior chamber IOL.

Intraocular lens implantation: Depending upon the state of the capsular bag and rhexis, IOL is implanted (Table 2.2).

In the bag: In the presence of a posterior capsule tear with good capsular bag, the IOL can be placed in the bag. Small PCR with no vitreous loss and good capsular bag, foldable IOL can be placed.

In the sulcus: If the rent is large, if the capsular rim is available, then the IOL can be placed in the sulcus. The rigid IOL can be placed in the sulcus in large PCR over the residual anterior capsular rim with Mc Person forceps holding the optic. The "chopstick technique" is another method of placing IOL in sulcus. In this new chopstick forceps namely, 'Agarwal- Katena forceps' (Figs 2.5A and B) is used for IOL implantation. This chopstick technique refers to the IOL being held between two flangs of the forceps. The advantage is the smooth placement of the IOL in the sulcus without excess manipulation. Moreover the IOL implantation is more controlled (Figs 2.6A to D) with the forceps as compared to other methods. Small PCR with no vitreous loss and good capsular bag, foldable IOL can be placed (Figs 2.7A and B). In eyes with intraoperative miosis with PCR, IOL can be implanted with the pupil expansion with "Agarwal's modified malyugin ring" method (Figs 2.8A and B). In this method,[10] a 6-0 polyglactic suture is placed in the leading scroll of the Malyugin ring and injected into the pupillary plane (Figs 2.9A and B). The end of the suture stays at the main port incision. Once in place, the ring produced a stable mydriasis of about 6.0 mm. Hereby IOL can implanted easily in the sulcus with visualization and this prevents the inadvertent dropping of the iris expander into the vitreous during intraoperative manipulation.

Deficient Posterior Capsule

Glued IOL[11,12,13] is easily performed in such cases with deficient posterior capsules. Scleral fixated posterior chamber lenses and anterior chamber IOLs[14,15] can also be implanted when the posterior capsule tear is large.

SEQUELAE AFTER POSTERIOR CAPSULAR RUPTURE

Vitreous traction: Incomplete vitrectomy can produce dynamic traction on the retina leading to retinal breaks.

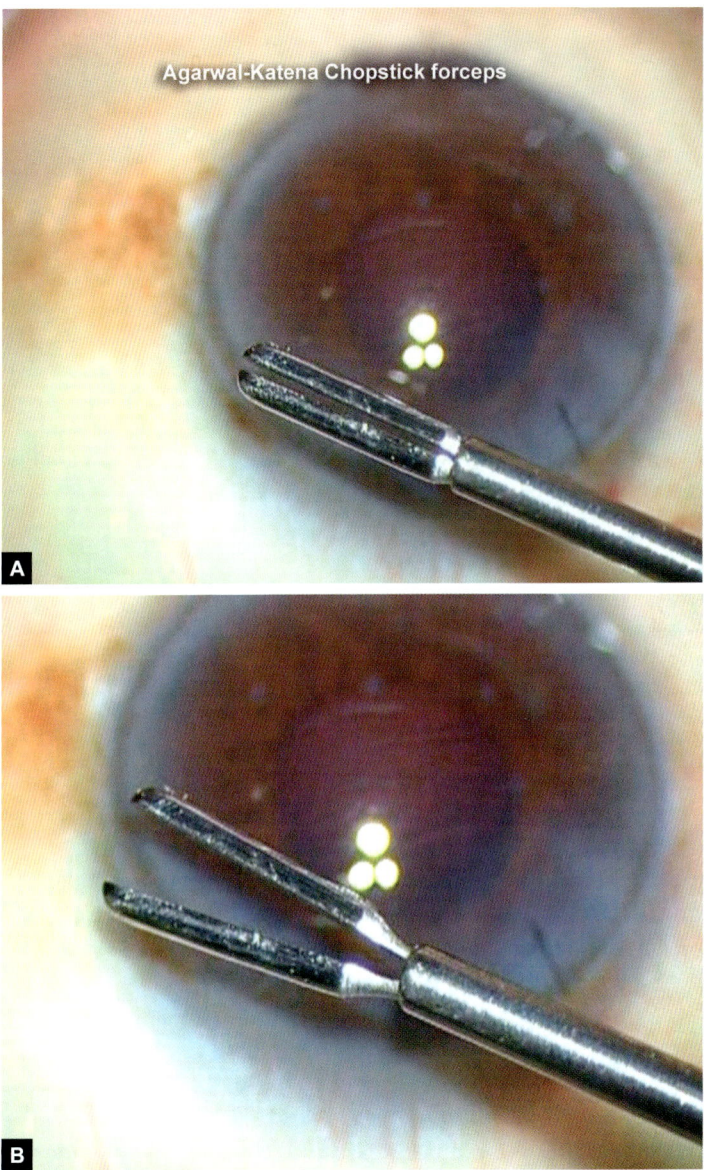

Figs 2.5A and B Photograph of an 'Agarwal- Katena' forceps. Reverse opening shown (left) (Katena, USA)

Retinal detachment: Undetected long standing vitreous traction progresses to retinal break and detachment.

Macular edema: Manipulation of vitreous will increase not only the traction transmitted to the retina but also the inflammation in the posterior segment, and the risk of macular edema.

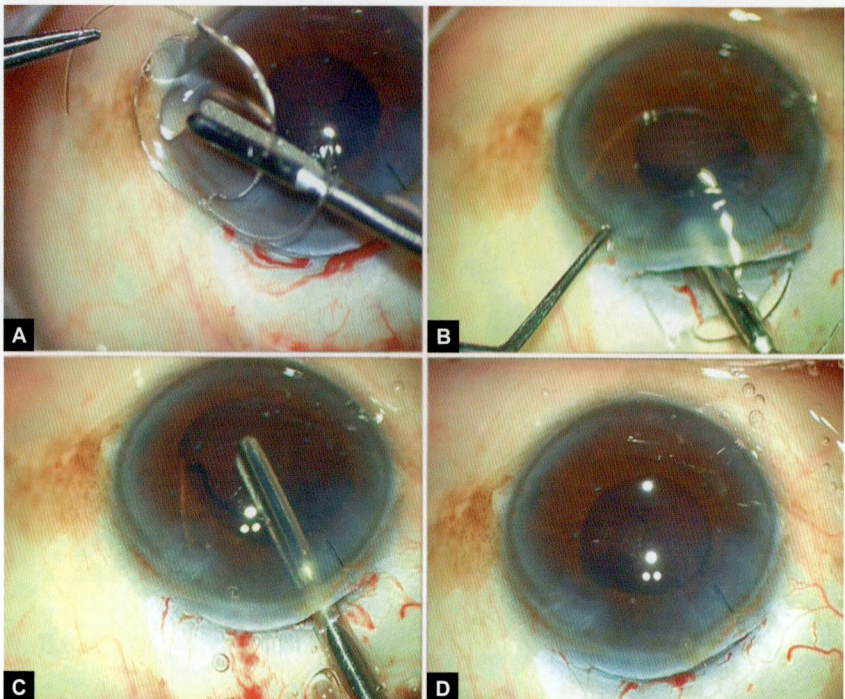

Figs 2.6A to D (A) The 6.5 mm PMMA rigid IOL being held between two flags of the forceps; (B) IOL is being introduced through the limbal incision; (C) IOL is positioned in the sulcus; (D) IOL is well centered

Vitritis: Over enthusiastic use of viscoelastic into the vitreous can lead to sterile inflammation. Dropped minimal residual cortex can also present with postoperative vitritis.

Intraocular lens related complications: Improperly placed IOL in the sulcus can lead to lens induced astigmatism and tilt.

CONCLUSION

The occurrence of a posterior capsule tear during cataract surgery is one of the most serious complications. It is important for a surgeon to diagnose the occurrence of a posterior capsule tear at an early stage to avoid further enlargement of the tear and associated vitreous complications. The primary goal of all the maneuvers is to remove the remaining nucleus, epinucleus, and as much cortex as possible without causing vitreoretinal traction.

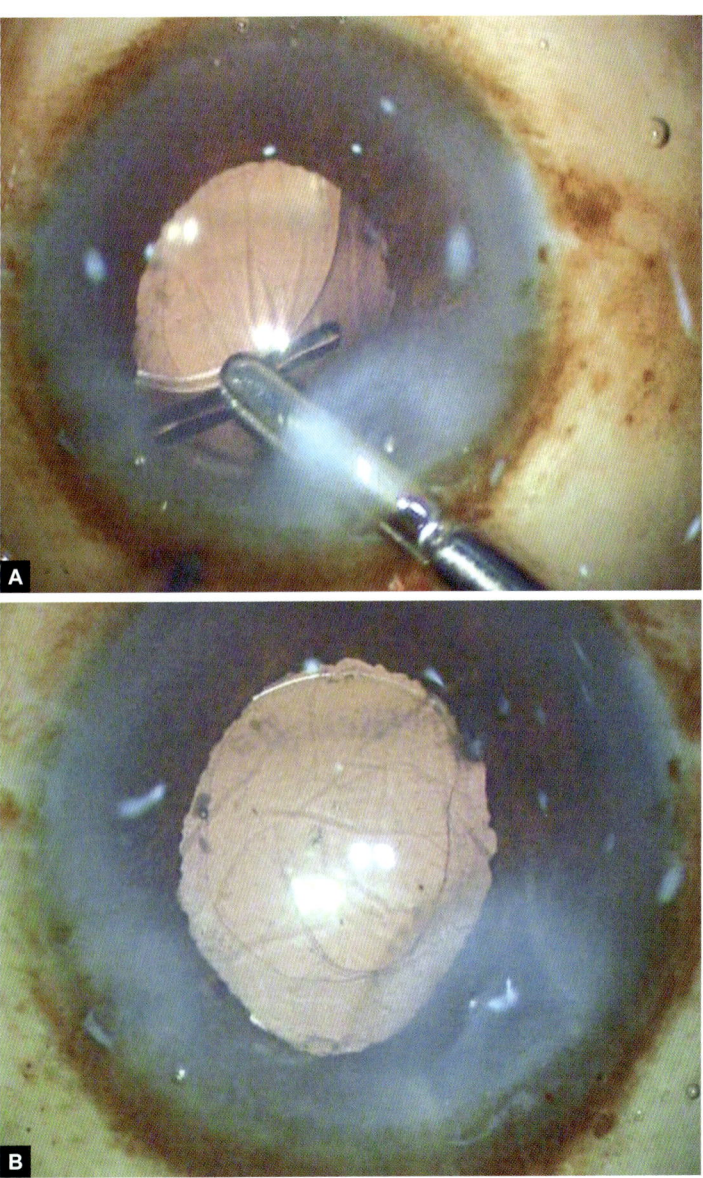

Figs 2.7A and B (A) Foldable IOL is placed with 'Agarwal–Katena' forceps into the sulcus; (B) IOL is well centered on the capsular rim

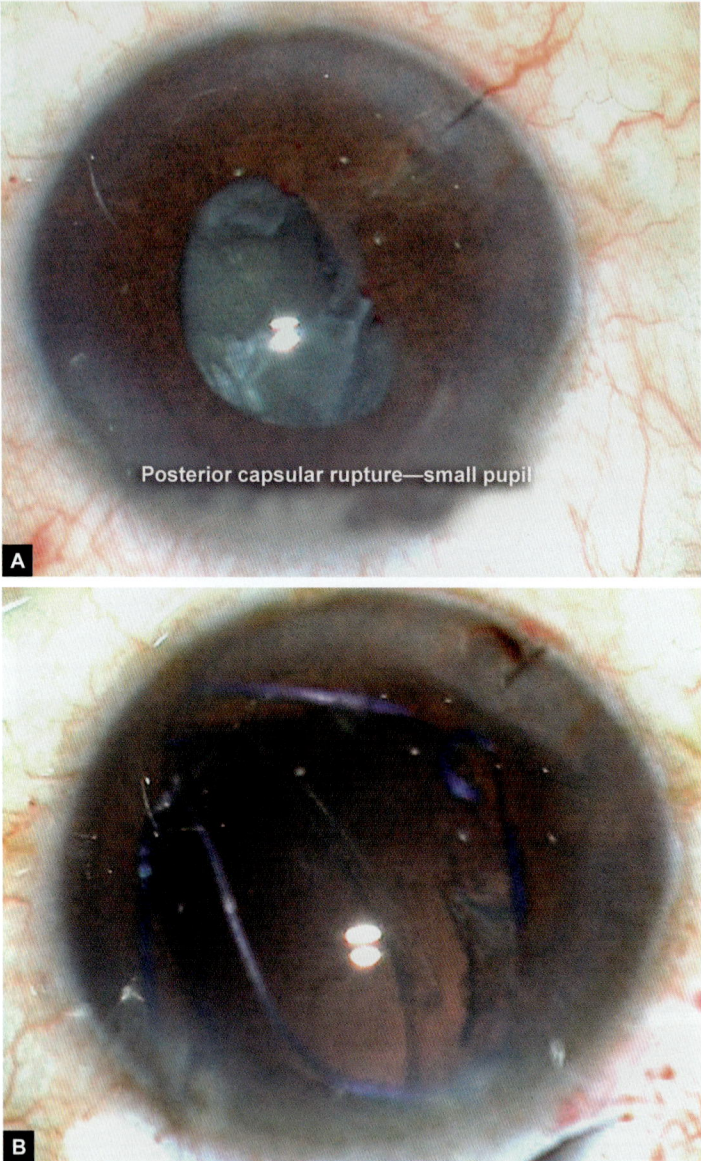

Figs 2.8A and B (A) Intraoperative miosis with posterior capsular tear; (B) Agarwal's modification of the Malyugin ring iris expansion: A 6-0 polyglactic vicryl suture passed in the leading scroll of the ring and injected. The end of the suture stays at the main port incision

Posterior Capsular Rupture

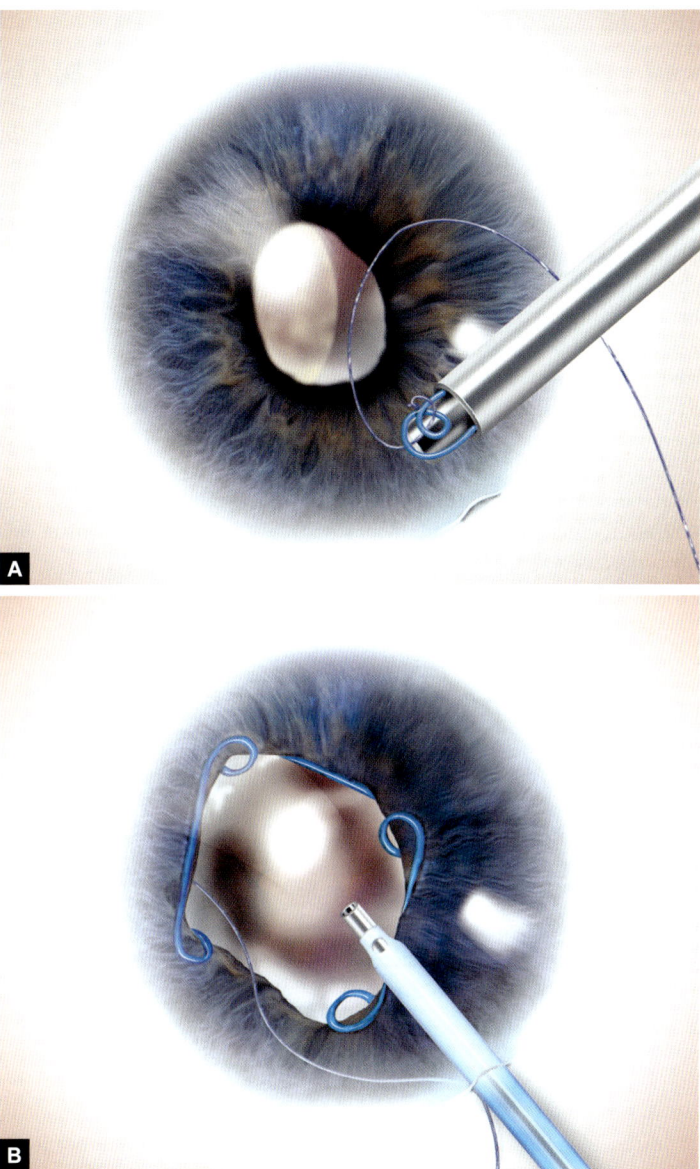

Figs 2.9A and B Illustration depicting the Agarwal modification of the Malyugin ring for cases with small pupil with a posterior capsular rupture. (A) 6/0 suture tied to the ring; (B) Malyugin ring is place in the pupil. The suture can be pulled at if the ring begins to fall into the vitreous

REFERENCES

1. Agarwal A. Phaco Nightmares; Conquering cataract catastrophes; Slack Inc, 2006, USA.
2. Agarwal S, Agarwal A, Agarwal A. Phacoemulsification –Two volume set; Third edn. Jaypee Brothers Medical Publishers; 2004, Delhi, India.
3. Fishkind W J. Facing Down the 5 Most Common Cataract Complications Review of Ophthalmology. October 2001.
4. Mulhern M, Kelly G, Barry P. Effects of posterior capsular disruption on the outcome of phacoemulsification surgery. Br J Ophthalmol. 1995;79:1133-7.
5. Osher RH, Cionni RJ. The torn posterior capsule: its intraoperative behaviour, surgical management and long term consequences. J Cataract Refract Surg. 1990;16:490-4.
6. Gimbel HV. Posterior capsular tears during phacoemulsification— causes, prevention and management. Eur J Refract Surg. 1990;2:63-9.
7. Vajpayee RB, Sharma N, Dada T, et al. Management of posterior capsule tears. Surv Ophthal 2001;45:473-88.
8. Peyman GA, Cheema R, Conway MD, Fang T. Triamcinolone acetonide as an aid to visualization of the vitreous and the posterior hyaloid during pars plana vitrectomy. Retina. 2000;20:554.
9. Burk SE, Da Mata AP, Snyder ME, Schneider S, Osher RH, Cionni RJ. Visualizing vitreous using Kenalog suspension. J Cataract Refract Surg. 2003;29:645.
10. Agarwal A, Malyugin B, Kumar DA, Jacob S, Agarwal A, Laks L. Modified Malyugin ring iris expansion technique in small-pupil cataract surgery with posterior capsule defect. J Cataract Refract Surg. 2008;34(5):724-6.
11. Agarwal A, Kumar DA, Jacob S, et al. Fibrin glue–assisted sutureless posterior chamber intraocular lens implantation in eyes with deficient posterior capsules. J Cataract Refract Surg. 2008;34:1433-8.
12. Agarwal A, Kumar DA, Prakash G, et al. Fibrin glue–assisted sutureless posterior chamber intraocular lens implantation in eyes with deficient posterior capsules [Reply to letter]. J Cataract Refract Surg. 2009;35:795-6.
13. Prakash G, Kumar DA, Jacob S, et al. Anterior segment optical coherence tomography-aided diagnosis and primary posterior chamber intraocular lens implantation with fibrin glue in traumatic phacocele with scleral perforation. J Cataract Refract Surg 2009;35:782-4.
14. Bleckmann H, Kaczmarek U. Functional results of posterior chamber lens implantation with scleral fixation. J Cataract Refract Surg. 1994;20:321-6.
15. Numa A, Nakamura J, Takashima M, Kani K. Long-term corneal endothelial changes after intraocular lens implantation. Anterior vs posterior chamber lenses Jpn J Ophthalmol 1993;37:78-87.

CHAPTER 3

Pars Plicata Anterior Vitrectomy: A Redefined Approach

Priya Narang, Amar Agarwal

INTRODUCTION

Posterior capsule rupture (PCR) while the nucleus is yet to be emulsified is a precipitous and intimidating complication that puts the surgeon on a high 'adrenaline rush'. A PCR is always an unwelcomed situation and is a cataract surgeon's nightmare. This complication is often further precipitated by the constriction of pupil and inability to do a proper vitrectomy as desired by the surgeon.

A limbal incision vitrectomy which is a preferred site by most of the anterior segment surgeons, often leads to the collapse of anterior chamber and an improper access to the lenticular matter trapped in the pupillary plane. Potential limitations of this approach include the fixed directionality of the instruments and cannula, which may lead to corneal distortion and poor visualization, and the fulcrum effect of the cannula may restrict the instrument movement too.

Pars plana has always been a favored choice of sclerotomy site for vitrectomy and retinal surgeries due to various reasons. In literature, limbal based and pars plana vitrectomy are the two well-defined methods of performing a thorough vitrectomy following a PCR. The idea to choose pars plicata as a route for performing a thorough anterior vitrectomy crept in from the technique of Glued IOL surgery; where a sclerotomy is made at the level of pars plicata followed by vitrectomy from the same site. Invariably, pars plicata site is an underutilized option for performing anterior vitrectomy. Surgical complications related to the insertion and removal of instruments through the pars plana incisions during vitrectomy has been well described. Retinal breaks and dialyses posterior to the sclerotomy are known to occur intraoperatively owing to the mechanical traction on anterior vitreous.

ANATOMIC CONSIDERATIONS

The ciliary body comprises of two parts: pars plicata and pars plana. About 1.5 mm from the limbus, pars plicata extends for about 2 mm and pars plana extends for about 4 mm up to ora serrata. The ciliary plexus lies at the root of iris and chance of hitting these blood vessels is high with pars plicata sclerotomy. On the other hand, vitreous base is located in the lower 2 mm of pars plana and improper sclerotomy done at this site can induce peripheral retinal tear, dialysis or sometimes a retinal detachment too if the fluid is kept '**ON**' during the introduction of infusion cannula.

Anatomically, a major arterial vascular circle is located at the root of iris and forms a complete ring around the peripheral border of the iris. A forceful entry at pars plicata should be avoided during sclerotomy and if resistance is encountered the probability of hitting the root of iris is very high.

Secondly, the vitreous is firmly attached to its neighboring tissues at peripheral retina, at the pars plana of the ciliary body and at the vitreous base. The vitreous base is a zone 3 to 4 mm wide which straddles the ora serrata. The collagen fibrils at the vitreous base are very dense and strongly adherent to the posterior pars plana and perioral retina. Any undue manipulation at this site can lead to peripheral retinal tear and dialysis which requires further management by a vitreoretinal surgeon.

The inhibition to use pars plana/pars plicata site creeps in from the idea of damaging the retina and disturbing the vitreous which can then inadvertently affect the final visual output. A major advantage of performing vitrectomy behind the pupillary plane is to provide a better fluidic seal, a better access to the retropupillary area and to the plane of the capsulorhexis following which the technique to adopt for an IOL implantation can be decided taking various factors into account.

In as early as 1990, pars plicata sclerotomy has been successfully reported to be helpful for repositioning a posteriorly dislocated IOL.[1] The pars plicata approach also has many advantages over the translimbal approach. The pars plicata is in the direct axis of the lens, allowing for more complete removal of lenticular material. In contrast to the limbal approach, the cornea is not manipulated during surgery. Deep visualization of the fundus is possible with a wide field lens of Volk, and lens fragments in the vitreous can be removed, thus preventing persistent inflammation postoperatively.

In our series of glued IOL surgery, sclerotomy is made at the level of pars plicata; approximately 1.5 mm away from the limbus just beneath the scleral flaps. The haptics of the IOL are externalized from these sclerotomy sites with a 25 gauge glued IOL forceps. In the review of complications profile of 486 eyes with rigid IOL, and 191 eyes with foldable IOL, posterior segment complications included macular edema (1.4%), retinal detachment (1%) and chronic vitritis (0.4%).[2]

These results suggest that pars plicata site can be taken advantage of and a thorough vitrectomy can be done through this site without the fear of damaging either the retina or the vitreous base.

SURGICAL TECHNIQUE

After the acknowledgment of PCR in a routine phacoemulsification procedure being done with corneal incision, the surgery is temporarily halted and anterior chamber is inflated with a dispersive ophthalmic viscosurgical device (OVD) from the side port incision before the withdrawal of phacoemulsification probe. The extent, position and the stage at which a PCR has occurred is taken into consideration. The main corneal incision is closed with a 10-0 suture and an anterior chamber maintainer/Trocar-cannula is introduced.

The site of sclerotomy can be chosen depending upon the primary incision for the cataract surgery and also on the location and extent of PCR and the retained cortical fragments. A small circumferential conjunctival peritomy incision 1.5 mm posterior to the limbus is fashioned and an entry with a microvitreoretinal (MVR) blade is made. The blade is inserted through the sclera, 1.5 mm posterior to the limbus with the direction of the blade obliquely downwards towards the mid-vitreous cavity. Alternatively, a trocar can also be used to create a sclerotomy wound (Fig. 3.1).

A 23 gauge vitrectomy cutter is introduced from this site (Fig. 3.2) and an adequate cutting rate with moderate amount of suction and flow rate is maintained and a thorough vitrectomy is done with better access and management of the vitreous and cortical fragments. Vitrectomy is performed under direct visualization to debulk the vitreous in the pupillary plane (Fig. 3.3). The anteriorly prolapsed vitreous is addressed through the posterior capsule

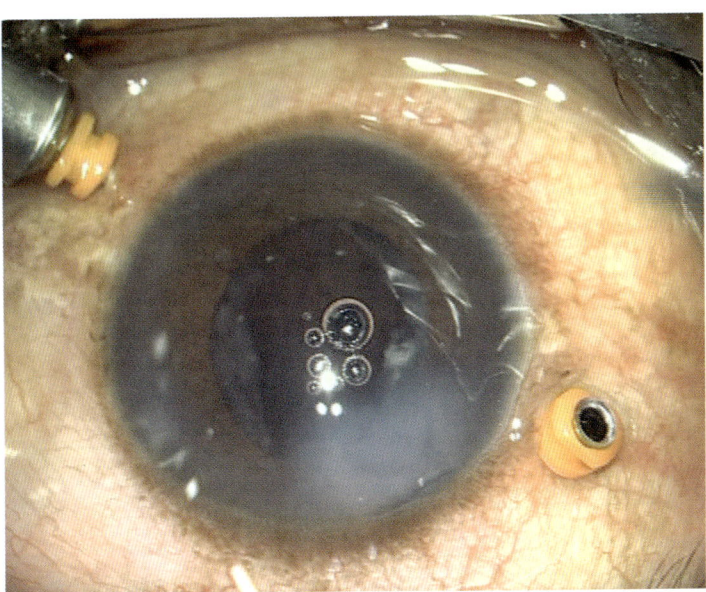

Fig. 3.1 Sclerotomy with trocar-cannula at pars plicata about 1.5 mm from the limbus

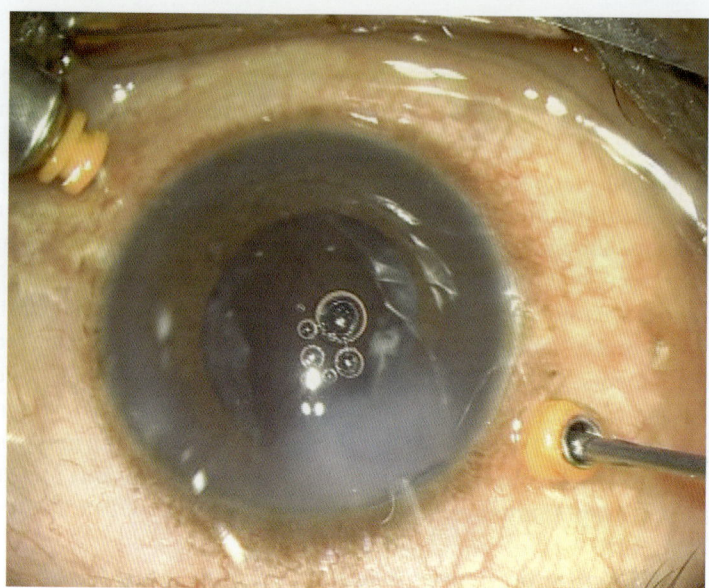

Fig. 3.2 A 23 gauge vitrectomy probe is being introduced from the pars plicata site

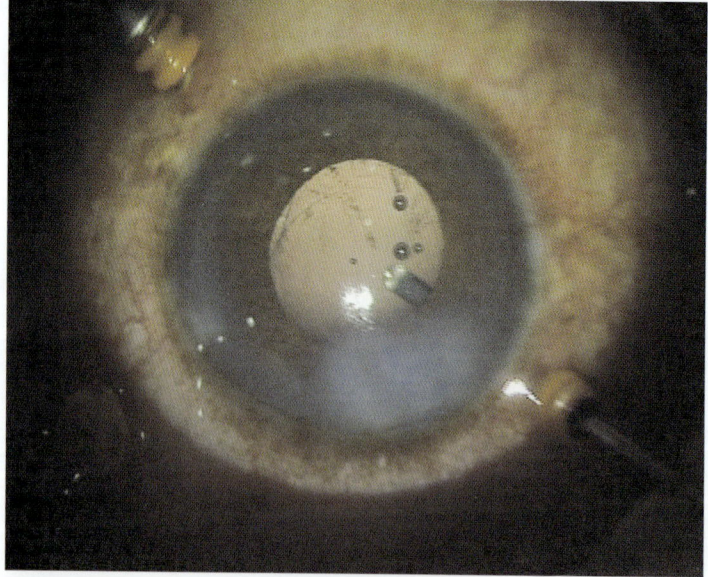

Fig. 3.3 Pars plicata vitrectomy is being done. Cortical matter cleared

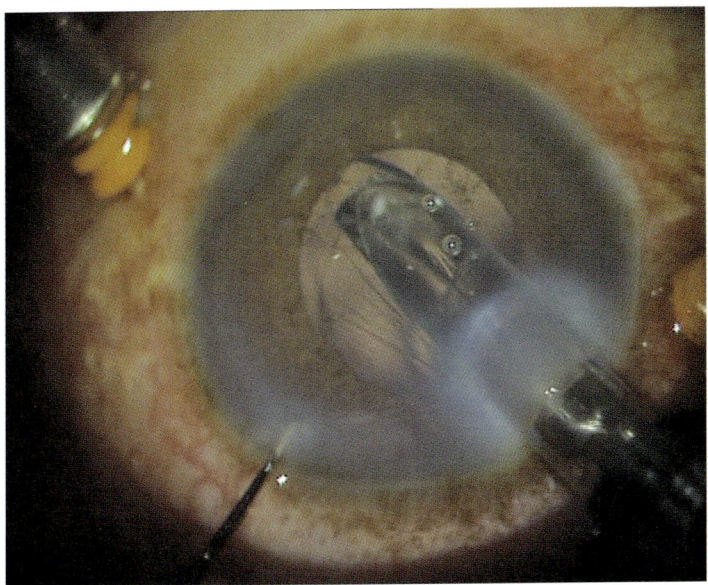

Fig. 3.4 A 3-piece foldable intraocular lens is being injected

tear. Precautions are taken to avoid extending the capsule tear and protecting the anterior capsulorhexis margin.

Triamcinolone acetonide can be used to visualize vitreous in the anterior chamber. Following the completion of vitrectomy, the cutter is removed and pressure is applied for wound closure. The capsular bag and residual capsule support are assessed to determine the final placement of an IOL. In cases of good sulcus support, a 3-piece foldable IOL is loaded and injected inside the eye (Fig. 3.4), which is then dialed into the sulcus. Stromal hydration is done and the wound is secured with 10-0 suture if necessary (Fig. 3.5).

PRECAUTIONS

A forceful entry at pars plicata should be avoided during sclerotomy. If resistance is encountered then the chances are that the surgeon is at the level of root of iris. A forceful entry at this juncture can lead to iridodialysis and also hyphema. The trocar or an MVR blade which is used to create a sclerotomy should be withdrawn and a fresh entry should be attempted slightly below the site of previous entry.

Surgical complications related to the insertion and removal of instruments through the pars plana incisions during vitrectomy have been well described.[3-5] Retinal breaks and dialyses posterior to the sclerotomies are known to occur intraoperatively owing to mechanical traction on the anterior vitreous. A peripheral retinal examination particularly at sclerotomy entry sites before

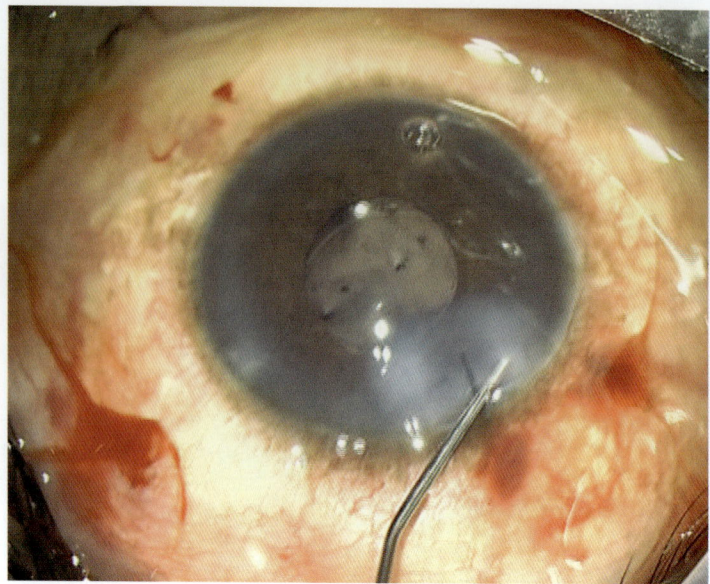

Fig. 3.5 Stable positioning of IOL on sulcus support

completion of surgery is advocated. Precautions which should be considered include minimizing instrumentation and the number of instrument changes, ensuring good vitreous clearance at sclerotomy sites, and avoiding vitreous incarceration. Multiple uses of disposable instruments, such as the vitrectomy cutter, may be associated with blunting, vitreoretinal traction, and therefore increased occurrence of retinal breaks. Ideally, single-use vitrectomy cutters should not be reused for this reason. The pars plicata approach has been used successfully in children with ROP.[6] An incision made in the pars plana of young children may increase the risk of retinal detachment. Because the pars plicata is further anterior from the vitreous base and ora serrata, the risk of retinal detachment is lessened.

DISCUSSION

This chapter represents and illustrates the surgical approach of pars plicata vitrectomy for phacoemulsification cases complicated by a PCR and residual cortical fragments.

Lensectomy and anterior vitrectomy via a pars plana or pars plicata approach is a suitable and safe method for treating cataract in children. Pars plana has always been a favored site for posterior vitrectomy in almost all cases as the surgical access through the pars plana requires entry approximately 3 to 4 mm behind the limbus to avoid trauma to the lens or to the retina. But, in cases of PCR, as the manipulation is at the level of lens and posterior capsule; a slightly anterior approach at the level of pars plicata is a suitable option as it offers protection and a safe margin against damaging the strong vitreal adhesions at the level of pars plana and vitreous base. Pars plana approach is not a reasonable idea for anterior vitrectomy because the pars plana entry has a risk of iatrogenic tears in the peripheral retina. In pediatric cases requiring vitrectomy, an age based placement of sclerotomy incision is taken into consideration to minimize both an inadvertent lens and retinal trauma. Sclerotomies are often placed more anteriorly in cases in which lens removal is anticipated, despite an otherwise morphologically normal posterior segment.

An MVR blade or a trocar cannula can be used to create the sclerotomy incision. The trocar-cannula system has an added advantage of obviating the need for conjunctival incision and providing a self-sealing wound.

The implantation of an acrylic hydrophobic 3-piece foldable IOL in the sulcus and in glued intrascleral IOL fixation preserves the advantages of a small-incision cataract surgery. The modified C-loop haptics of the IOL improves stabilization at the sulcus and applies even, equal tension to the adjacent tissues and the 6.0 mm optic diameter lowers the risk of symptomatic postoperative decentration. Bimanual vitrectomy is preferred in all the cases as a separate infusion prevents the cortical fragments from being pushed away during the chewing up process.

Apart from this, in cases of pars plicata vitrectomy done for all age groups, we did not come across any major complication and had a very gratifying and a favorable outcome. An extensive vitrectomy also prevents pupillary block glaucoma resulting from a vitreous prolapsed into the anterior chamber. Lastly, the vitreous is removed without trauma to the iris, which has been a suspected cause of cystoid macula edema.[7] For anterior segment surgeons who are reluctant to make a pars plana incision following a PCR, this site can be explored and advantage can be availed.

REFERENCES

1. Lyons CJ, Steele AD. Report of a repositioned posteriorly dislocated intraocular lens via pars plicata sclerotomy. J Cataract Refract Surg. 1990;16(4):509-11.
2. Kumar DA, Agarwal A. Glued intraocular lens: a major review on surgical technique and results. Curr Opin Ophthalmol. 2013;24:21-9.
3. Aaberg TM. Pars plana vitrectomy for diabetic tractional retinal detachment. Ophthalmology. 1981;88:639-42.
4. Faulborn J, Conway BP, Machemer R. Surgical complications of pars plana vitreous surgery. Ophthalmology. 1978;85:116-25.
5. Machemer R. A new concept for vitreous surgery: II. Surgical technique and complications. Am J Ophthalmol. 1972;74:1022-33.
6. Gonzales CR, Boshra J, Schwartz SD. 25-gauge pars plicata vitrectomy for stage 4 and 5 retinopathy of prematurity. Retina. 2006;26:42-6.
7. Grossman SA, Peyman G. Long-term visual results after pars plicata lensectomy-vitrectomy for congenital cataracts. Br J Ophthalmol. 1988;72:601-6.

CHAPTER 4

Sleeveless Phacotip Assisted Levitation of Dropped Nucleus

Priya Narang, Amar Agarwal

INTRODUCTION

Dropped nucleus is a serious complication of phacoemulsification as it causes severe morbidity to the patient if not handled properly. It can occur at any stage varying from hydrodissection, rotation of nucleus, chopping or trenching to irrigation/aspiration. Management of sinking nucleus in early stages is quite a tricky trap as a large chunk is yet to be emulsified. The vitreous often serves as a barrier to prevent the entire nucleus from sinking and resting on the bed of retina. But this barrier is not very effective in high myopes and old patients as the vitreous is liquefied. A brisk response from the surgeon without getting panicked is all that is needed at this juncture.

Management can differ depending on the location of the chunk in the vitreous. One of the various techniques employed for nucleus in anterior vitreous cavity is the posterior-assisted levitation where a metal spatula is inserted through pars plana incision, and the fragments are manipulated into the anterior chamber. In 'Viscoat PAL' technique; the Viscoat is injected behind the partially descended fragment through pars plana, where it can provide a safety net to the descending nucleus. The nuclear fragment is then levitated into the anterior chamber. A chopstick technique is also employed by some surgeons wherein the nuclear fragment is trapped between two sinskey hooks and is then levitated in the anterior chamber. Nuclear fragments in the mid-vitreous cavity and beyond should be handled by vitreoretinal surgeons as further 'fishing' into the vitreous cavity is not recommended.

In 1999, we started a technique for levitating dropped nucleus and termed it as FAVIT. 'FAVIT' technique — FAVIT for 'fallen vitreous,' as the name describes a method to remove lens fragments that have 'fallen' into the 'vitreous.' This technique evolved and eventually improved with the advancements in ophthalmology to take the current shape; making it more safe, easy and reliable to perform. It is now known as sleeveless phacotip assisted levitation of dropped nucleus (SPAL).

SURGICAL TECHNIQUE

Following a nucleus drop, a standard 23 gauge 3-port pars plana vitrectomy incisions are framed (Fig. 4.1). An anterior vitrectomy is done and cortical matter lying in the anterior chamber or sulcus area is removed which improves the visualization of the vitreous cavity (Fig. 4.2). The initial step is complete removal of the vitreous to prevent traction on the retina from subsequent maneuvers. A thorough vitrectomy is performed and all the vitreous adhesions surrounding the retained lens fragment and the retinal surface are released using the vitrectomy probe (Fig. 4.3). A reinverter system with VOLK wide field lens is used for adequate visualization of the posterior chamber. Triamcinolone injection can be used to facilitate the staining of the vitreous strands at this stage.

After completion of posterior vitrectomy, the vitrectomy probe is replaced with the sleeveless phacoemulsification probe. Suction only mode is used on the phacoemulsification probe to lift the lens off the retina and hold it while it is repositioned into the anterior chamber. Suction is generated when the phacotip is close to the nucleus in order to avoid any entrapment of the vitreous strand into the lumen (Fig. 4.4). A small burst of ultrasonic energy is applied in the mid-vitreal cavity to embed the phacotip into the elevated lens fragment to improve nucleus stabilization, and then the entire fragment is lifted anteriorly and brought into the mid-pupillary plane (Fig. 4.5). The instrument in the nondominant hand is also used at the same time to guide the lens fragment above the iris plane and into the anterior chamber.

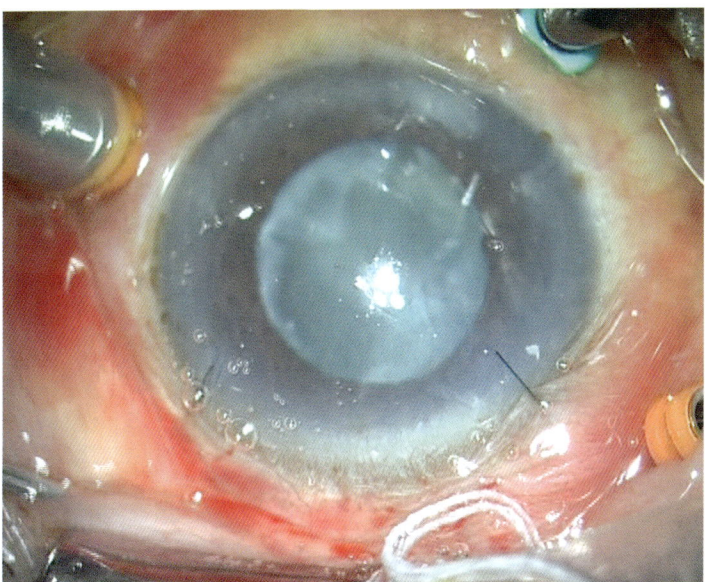

Fig. 4.1 Intraoperative dropped nucleus. Standard 3-port 23 G vitrectomy incisions framed

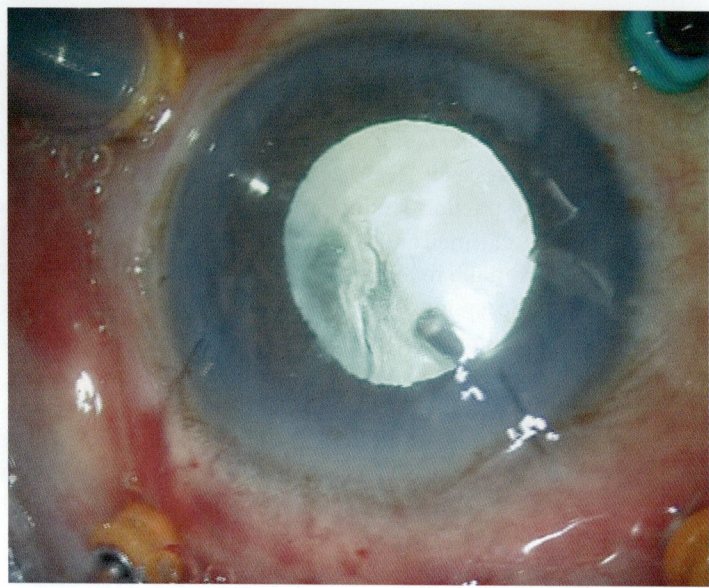

Fig. 4.2 Vitrectomy probe introduced to perform thorough anterior vitrectomy to enhance the visualization of the posterior segment

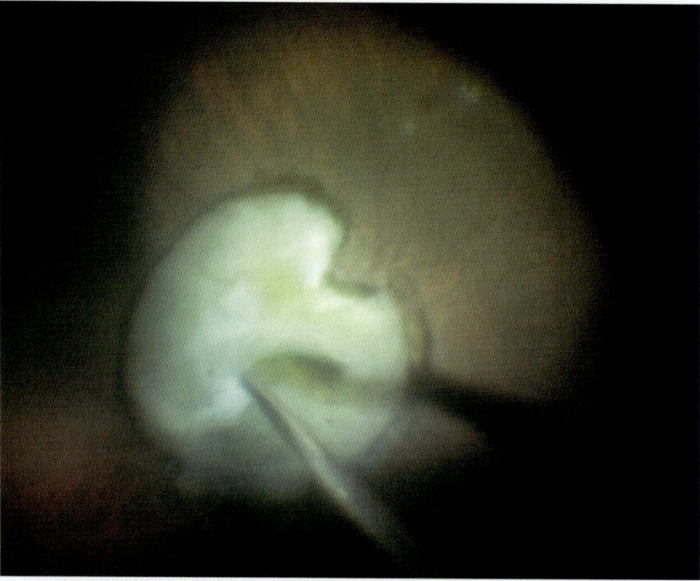

Fig. 4.3 Posterior segment vitrectomy is being done to release all vitreolenticular adhesions

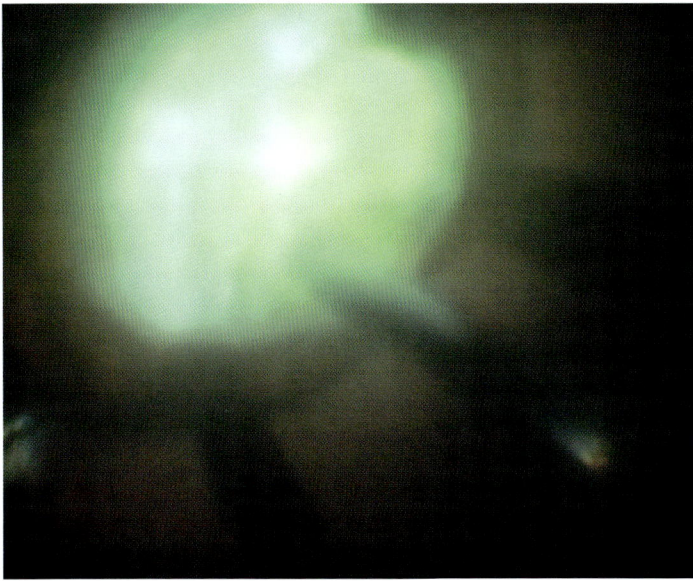

Fig. 4.4 Sleeveless phaco probe introduced and embedded in the nucleus with a short burst of energy

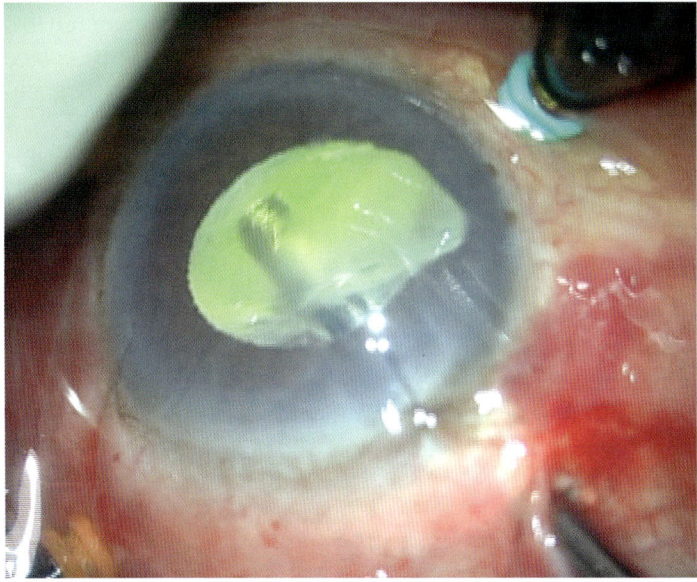

Fig. 4.5 The nuclear fragment levitated into the anterior chamber

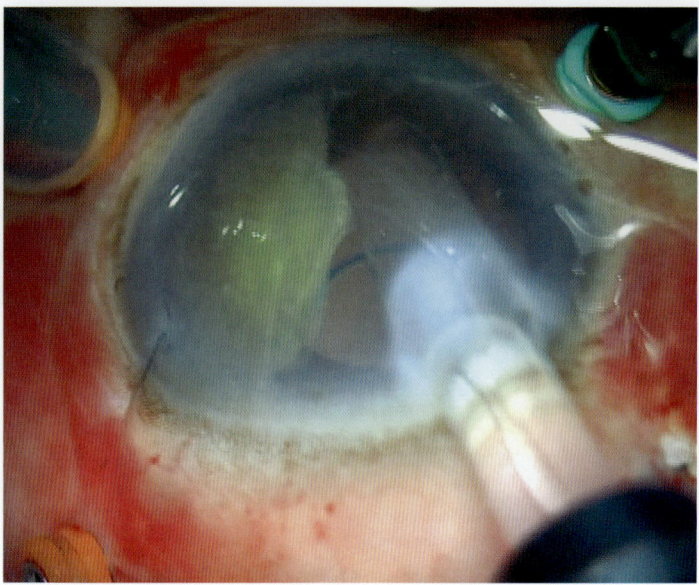

Fig. 4.6 A 3-piece foldable IOL is being injected beneath the nuclear fragment as in IOL scaffold technique

Upon levitation of the nucleus into the anterior chamber, the phaco probe is withdrawn. The nucleus can then be removed using either an IOL scaffold technique[1,2] (Figs 4.6 to 4.8) or an extra capsular extraction by enlarging the corneal incision. In cases of inadequate sulcus support, glued IOL scaffold[3] can also be performed.

Adequate examination of the posterior segment is done to ensure no cortical fragment is left in vitreous cavity (Fig. 4.9).

DISCUSSION

Dropped nucleus during phacoemulsification procedure poses a surgical challenge for surgeons. Pars plana vitrectomy is often used to address this complication but it is limited by the size of the cutter tip, vacuum, and cutting rate when hard nuclear fragments are involved. An ultrasonic fragmatome is often used to overcome this limitation. The fragmatome is the conventional ultrasound instrument for pars plana lensectomy; however, it needs a special handpiece and software which may not always be available. In addition, retinal damage or detachment can result from the transmission of ultrasonic waves through dislocated nuclear fragments located on the retina.[4] To prevent such damage, perfluorocarbon liquid (perfluoro-n-octane) (PFCL) have been used to block ultrasonic wave transmission to the retina. Ocular toxicity due to retained PFCL, including uncontrolled intraocular pressure,[5] corneal epithelial toxicity[6]

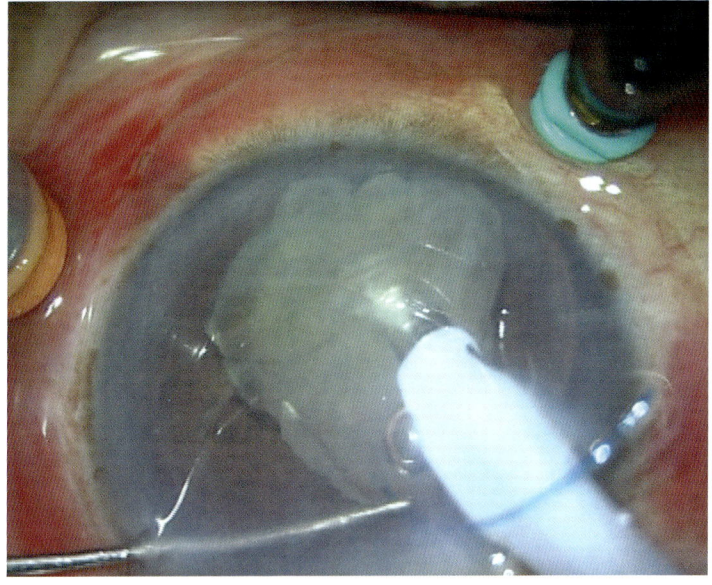

Fig. 4.7 Nucleus emulsified with phacoemulsification

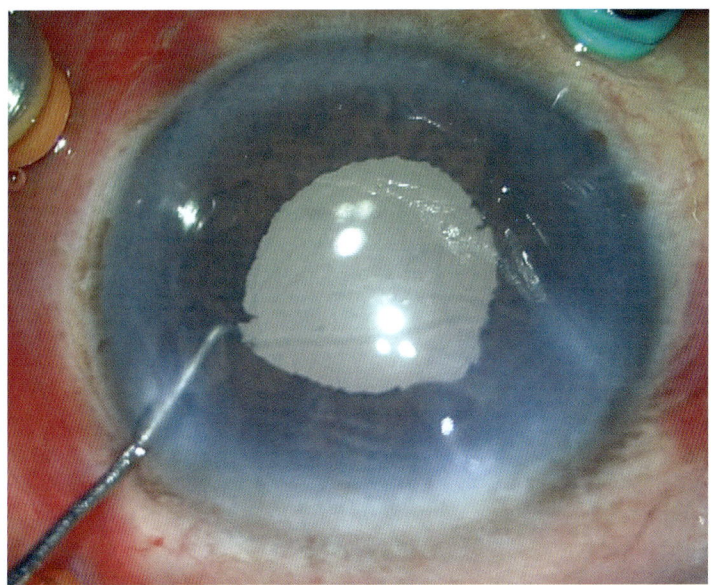

Fig. 4.8 Sulcus placed IOL is stable

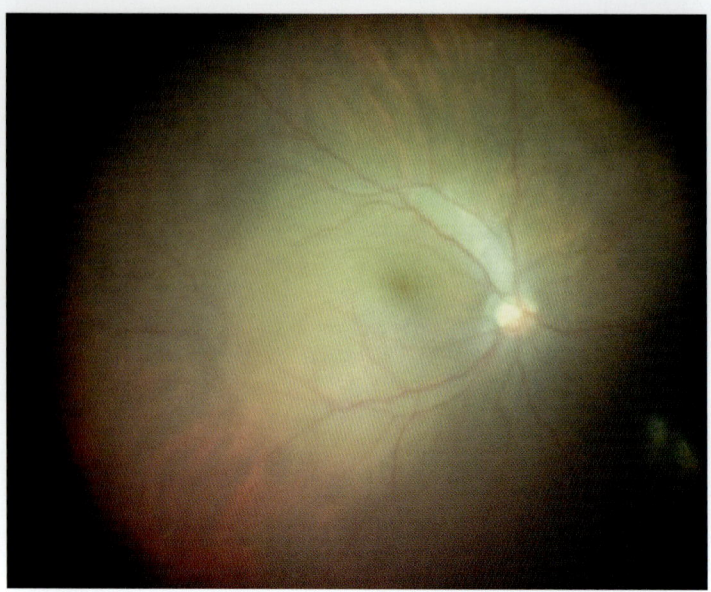

Fig. 4.9 Posterior segment examination shows no nuclear remnant

and decreased focal sensitivity of the retina[7] has been reported. *In vitro* study showed that PFCL is directly toxic to human retinal pigment epithelial cells when exposed to the cells for 7 days.[8]

In the SPAL technique, there is no strong intravitreal fluid current or inadvertent suction of residual vitreous gel resulting from the larger port of the phaco needle. The vacuum is generated when the phacotip is close to the dropped nucleus. Having a good hold of the lens material at the tip is crucial. A moderate amount of vacuum setting is enough to lift the nucleus adequately into the mid-vitreous cavity; followed by initiation of phaco power for adequate embedment. The advantage of holding the nucleus with a sleeveless phacotip enables a firm grip and the nucleus does not tend to fall back into the vitreous cavity. The firmly embedded nucleus is then easy to levitate into the anterior chamber. The recommended technique for employing ultrasound energy in the vitreous cavity is to lift the nucleus fragment away from the retinal surface by aspiration in the mid/anterior vitreous cavity, thereby limiting exposure of the posterior pole to ultrasound energy.[9] In addition, no excessive heat is generated at the incision site as the duration for which phaco energy used is minimal. Ordinary phacoemulsification needle have different lengths. A standard phaco needle is shorter than the fragmatome (23.2 mm versus 26.6 mm);[10] but we did not encounter any problem with nucleus engagement and embedment in our study. The grip achieved with the phaco needle is quite adequate and the nucleus does not tend to slip or fall back when trying to levitate in the anterior chamber; even when it comes in contact with adjacent tissues like iris. If the nucleus is nearly intact and is wider than the capsulotomy, it cannot physically move more anterior than the anterior capsule, because the latter acts as a barrier. In our series of patients, we did not encounter this hindrance.

The eyes in which the dropped nucleus has been removed require proper optical correction. Simultaneous IOL implantation and removal of a dropped nucleus is a benefit in these cases. After levitating the nucleus in anterior chamber, the IOL scaffold technique[1,2] was performed. In these cases with soft to moderate nucleus; a 3-piece foldable IOL when injected beneath the nuclear fragment, acts as a scaffold and prevents the nucleus from dropping back into the vitreous cavity. For dense nuclei, the corneal incision is enlarged and the nucleus is removed; alternatively a scleral tunnel can also be fashioned to remove the nucleus. This is followed by IOL implantation either in the sulcus or a glued intrascleral fixation of IOL[11] in cases with inadequate sulcus support. In cases with both inadequate iris and sulcus support, an IOL scaffold procedure cannot be done. In such cases, glued IOL scaffold[3] procedures can be performed, where initially glued IOL is done which fixes the IOL in place and this IOL in turn acts as a scaffold and prevents the nucleus from slipping into the vitreous cavity. The nucleus is then safely emulsified in the anterior chamber. SPAL technique eliminates the need to emulsify the nucleus in the vitreous cavity and its subsequent complications. In addition, no special instrument is required to perform SPAL. The technique when coupled with IOL scaffold, further enhances the visual outcome as it also provides all the advantages of a closed chamber corneal incision cataract surgery.

REFERENCES

1. Kumar DA, Agarwal A, Prakash G, et al. IOL scaffold technique for posterior capsular rupture. J Refract Surg. 2012;28:314-5.
2. Narang P, Agarwal A, Kumar DA, et al. Clinical outcomes of intraocular scaffold lens surgery. A one year study. Ophthalmology. 2013;120:2442-8.
3. Agarwal A, Jacob S, Agarwal A, Narasimhan S, Kumar DA, Agarwal A. Glued intraocular lens scaffolding to create an artificial posterior capsule for nucleus removal in eyes with posterior capsule tear and insufficient iris and sulcus support. J Cataract Refract Surg. 2013;39:32.
4. Movshovich A, Berrocal M, Chang S. The protective properties of liquid perflurocarbons in phacofragmentation of dislocated lenses. Retina. 1994;14:457-62.
5. Foster RE, Smiddy WS, Alfonso EC, Parrish RK. Secondary glaucoma associated with retained perfluorophenanthrene. Am J Ophthalmol. 1994;118:253-5.
6. Ramaesh K, Bhagat S, Wharton SB, Singh J. Corneal epithelial toxic effects and inflammatory response to perflurocarbon liquid. Arch Ophthalmol. 1999;117:1411-3.
7. Tewari A, Eliott D, Singh CN, Garcia-Valenzuela E, Ito Y, Abrams GW. Changes in retinal sensitivity from retained subretinal perflurocarbon liquid. Retina. 2009;29:248-50.

8. Inoue M, Iriyama A, Kadonosono K, Tamaki Y, Yanagi Y. Effects of perflurocarbon liquids and silicone oil on human retinal pigment epithelial cells and retinal ganglion cells. Retina. 2009;29:677-81.
9. Rofagha S, Bhisitkul RB. Management of retained lens fragments in complicated cataract surgery. Curr Opin Ophthalmol 2011;22:137-40.
10. Imai M, Iijima H, Takeda N. Intravitreal phacoemulsification with pars plana vitrectomy and posterior chamber intraocular lens suture fixation for dislocated crystalline lenses. J Cataract Refract Surg. 2001;27(11):1724-8.
11. Agarwal A, Kumar DA, Jacob S, Baid C, Agarwal A, Srinivasan S. Fibrin glue-assisted sutureless posterior chamber intraocular lens implantation in eyes with deficient posterior capsules. J Cataract Refract Surg. 2008;34:1433-8.

CHAPTER 5

Sleeveless Extrusion Cannula for Levitation of Dropped Intraocular Lens

Ashvin Agarwal, Priya Narang, Amar Agarwal

INTRODUCTION

Dislocated intraocular lens (IOL) in to the posterior chamber have always been a cause of concern and a known complication following a posterior capsule rupture. Improper sulcus fixation, dislocation/subluxation of the IOL bag complex or improper judgment about the integrity of posterior capsule intraoperatively, often lead to this complicated scenario. Dislocation of IOL not only makes the patient aphakic but can also cause complication related with dropped IOL. It is therefore mandatory to explant or reposition the IOL which in itself has its own complications and requires a major vitreoretinal intervention.

Various methods and techniques have been described to lift the dropped IOLs. Grasping instruments like retinal forceps have been used in the past but they run the risk of damaging the retina during the process of lifting the IOL. Perflurocarbons too have been used to facilitate the lifting and help in floating the IOL[1], so that it can be easily picked up. Santos et al[2] proposed the use of silicon tip aspiration cannula connected to the vitreotome. Olson et al[3] devised a special suction based grasping cup that could lift the IOL. Fragmatome tip has also been described to levitate posteriorly dislocated IOLs by applying suction.[4]

Extrusion cannula has been extensively used for drainage of subretinal fluid (SRF) by posterior segment surgeons. The flexible sleeve of the extrusion cannula helps to reach the subretinal space effectively. In our practice, we use extrusion cannula without sleeves for levitating dropped IOLs. Removal of the sleeve gives a wider area for adherence and subsequent creation of effective suction to the intraocular lens.

SURGICAL TECHNIQUE

After a standard three port pars plana vitrectomy procedure (Fig. 5.1) and clearance of all the vitreolenticular adhesions, the sleeveless extrusion cannula is connected to the vacuum of the vitreotome. Occluding the IOL before completing

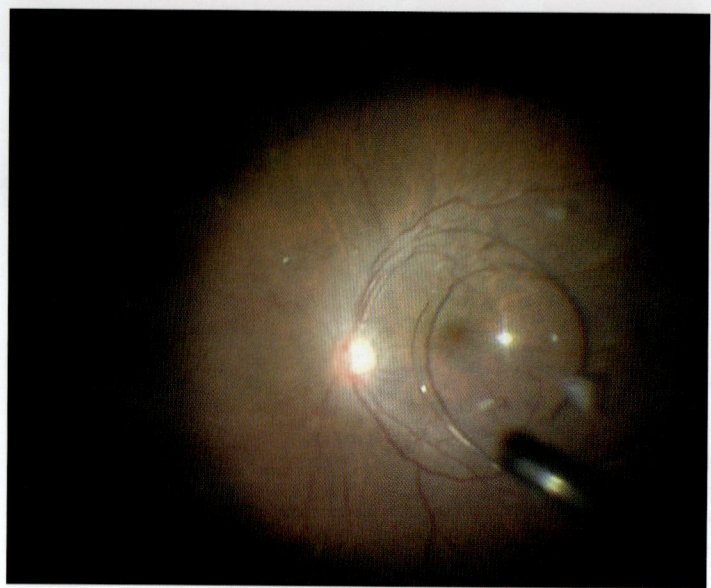

Fig. 5.1 Vitrectomy is being done to remove all the vitreolenticular adhesions

the vitrectomy is avoided to minimize the risk of peripheral retinal breaks due to trapping of the vitreous in the lumen of the cannula.

As the IOL rests flat on the retina, the sleeveless extrusion cannula is made to face the center of the optic and suction is initiated to allow a firm grasp (Fig. 5.2). Addressing the IOL with extrusion cannula without sleeves gives a larger surface area to be adhered to the IOL. The suction can be dynamically controlled with the foot pedal. The IOL is lifted from the surface of the retina and is brought into the anterior vitreous (Fig. 5.3) in the mid-pupillary area. The IOL is grasped by the end opening forceps introduced from the corneal incision under direct visualization through the microscope; the extrusion cannula is then removed as the forceps grasps the IOL (Fig. 5.4). The surgeon then proceeds to remove, reposition, or exchange the IOL, depending on the status of the capsulorhexis rim and the type of IOL in each individual case. The retinal periphery is checked 360° with scleral indentation to rule out any retinal breaks.

DISCUSSION

A dislocated IOL can cause complications such as decreased vision, monocular diplopia, glare, hyphema, iritis, secondary glaucoma, corneal decompensation, cystoid macular edema (CME), and peripheral retinal traction and subsequent retinal detachment.[5] The complications associated with dislocated IOLs like

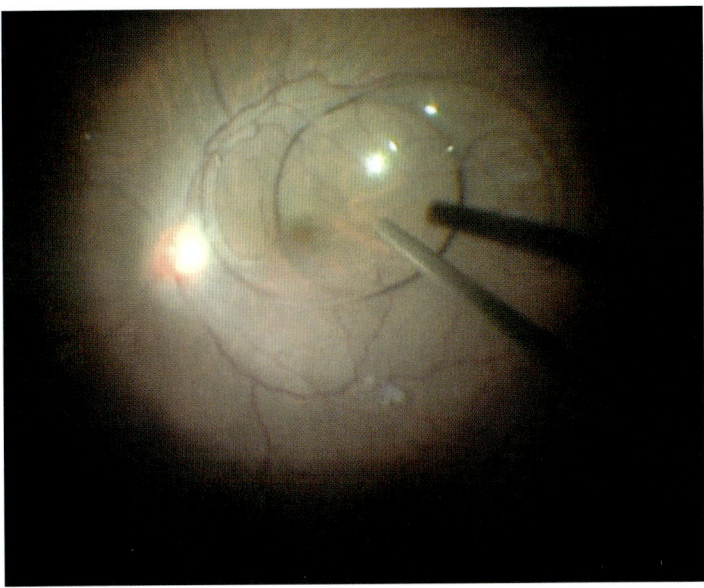

Fig. 5.2 Sleeveless extrusion cannula is introduced and is made to face the optic of the intraocular lens (IOL)

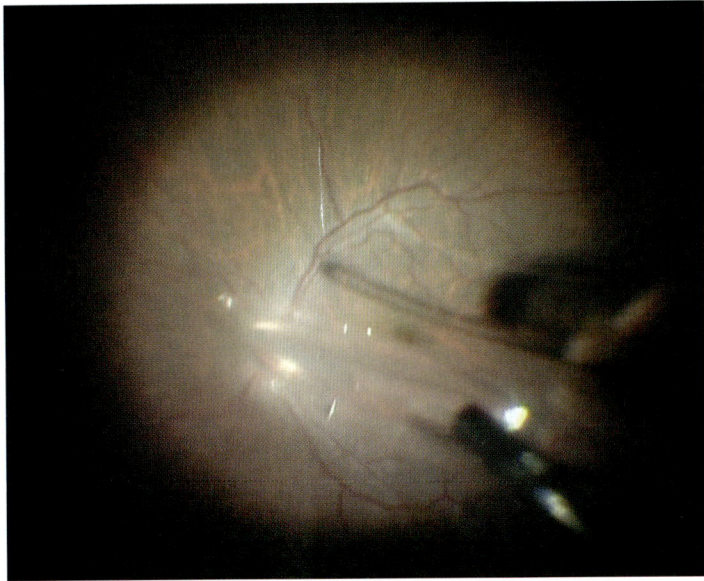

Fig. 5.3 The suction is initiated and the IOL is levitated into the midpupillary area

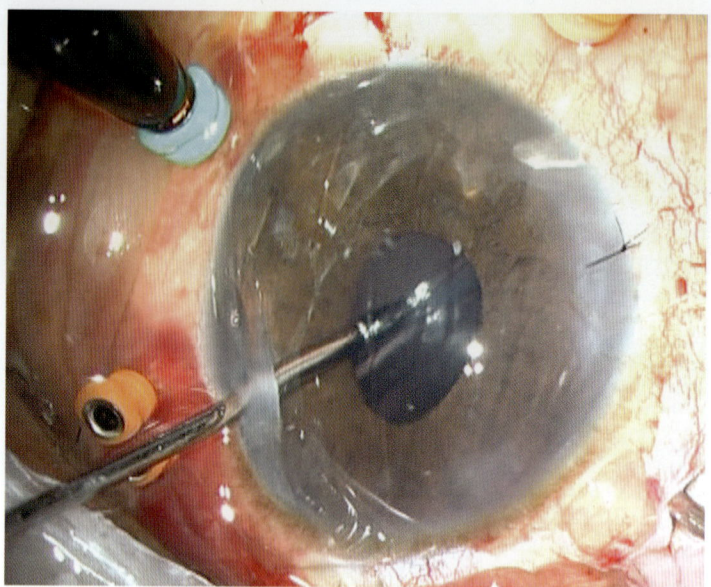

Fig. 5.4 The IOL is grasped by an end-opening forceps

CME, corneal edema, glaucoma, and intraocular inflammation are often difficult to differentiate from consequences of the initial complicated cataract surgery. In our limited series of cases, we did not come across any major complication; probably as the effective time interval between the original cataract surgery and the dislocated IOL levitation was minimal. This highlights that the levitation technique with sleeveless extrusion cannula is an effective method although the final visual outcome can be affected by many variables in a complicated cataract surgery.

The advantage with this procedure is that no special instrument is required for the surgery. Care should be taken to initiate vacuum when the cannula is close to the IOL. This helps to prevent any accidental trapping of the vitreous strand in to the lumen of the extrusion cannula. Another advantage is that the chances of damaging the retina while levitating the IOL are almost nullified unlike the grasping instruments used in the vitreous cavity. In our experience, it allows safe and easy access to the dropped IOL with minimal surgical interventions.

REFERENCES

1. Lewis H, Sanchez G. The use of perfluorocarbon liquids in the repositioning of posteriorly dislocated intraocular lenses. Ophthalmology. 1993;100:1055-9.
2. Santos A, Roig-Melo EA. Management of posteriorly dislocated intraocular lens: a new technique. Ophthalmic Surg Lasers. 2001;32:260-2.

3. Olson JL, Montoya RV, Erlanger M, Mackenzie D. Management of a dislocated intraocular lens with a suction-based grasping tool. J Cataract Refract Surg. 2013;39:154-7.
4. Jorge R, Siqueira RC, Cardillo JA, Costa RA. Fragmatome lifting: surgical option for intraocular lens and foreign body removal. Ophthalmic Surg Lasers Imaging. 2005;36:261-4.
5. Brod RD, Flynn HW Jr, Clarkson JG, Blankenship GW. Management options for retinal detachment in the presence of a posteriorly dislocated intraocular lens. Retina. 1990;10:50-6.

SECTION II

Glued Intraocular Lens and Intraocular Lens Scaffold

CHAPTER **6**

Glued Intrascleral Haptic Fixation of Intraocular Lens (Glued IOL)

Ashvin Agarwal, Amar Agarwal

INTRODUCTION

Posterior capsular rent (PCR) can occur in the early learning curve in phacoemulsification.[1-15] Intraoperative dialysis or a large PCR prevents IOL implantation in the capsular bag. Implantation of an IOL in the sulcus is possible in cases of adequate anterior capsular support. The first glued PCIOL implantation in an eye with a deficient capsule was done on 14th December 2007. In eyes with inadequate anterior capsular rim and deficient posterior capsule, the new technique of IOL implantation is the fibrin glue assisted sutureless IOL implantation with scleral tuck.[3-7] Since 2007, a large number of cases have been done with this technique. The technique has also evolved since then and extended its application to many different scenarios and as part of combined surgeries. The scleral tuck and intrascleral haptic fixation of a PCIOL was first started by Gabor Scharioth from Germany.[8] Maggi had previously done a sutureless scleral fixation of a special IOL.[9]

WHITE TO WHITE MEASUREMENT

One should always measure the corneal white to white (WTW) diameter. If the horizontal WTW is about 11 mm then a horizontal glued IOL can be performed. This means the flaps can be made at 3 and 9 O'clock positions. If the WTW is more then it is better to do a vertical glued IOL which means the scleral flaps are made at 12 and 6 O'clock positions. The reason this is performed is that the vertical cornea will always be shorter than the horizontal, so one will have more haptic to tuck and glue. This idea was suggested by *Jeevan Ladi* from India.

SURGICAL TECHNIQUE

Conjunctival Peritomy

If one is performing a manual nonphaco technique or a nonfoldable glued IOL implantation, then it is better to have the superior rectus being caught and

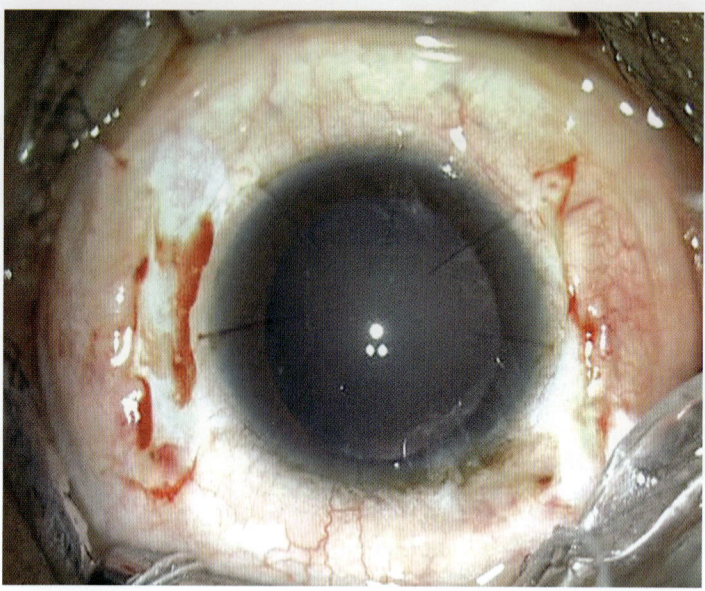

Fig. 6.1 Conjunctival peritomy and scleral marking done

secured as exposure is better. In such cases, one should prepare the conjunctival peritomy in the areas where the scleral flaps are to be made. Adequate but not over excessive cautery should be done to stop any bleeding vessels (Fig. 6.1).

Scleral Marking

It is imperative that the scleral flaps are 180 degrees apart. If not, then the IOL will be decentered. For this reason, it is better to use a scleral marker which creates marks on the cornea to see that the scleral flaps created are diagonally opposite (Fig. 6.1).

Scleral Flap Preparation

The size of the flaps should be 2.5 mm by 2.5 mm with the base at the limbus. Too large a flap is not ideal as the haptic has to traverse a longer distance to get tucked. There are many ways by which the scleral flap can be prepared just like one prepares a trabeculectomy flap. Sometimes it is cumbersome to create these flaps as one might have to use the nondominant hand. A simple way by which we perform the scleral flaps is to first use a knife to create a mark on the sclera to up to half thickness. One should be careful not to make it too deep or too shallow. Once the marks are made, then one should take the hockey flap dissector (same one which one uses to make a scleral tunnel) and pass it from one end of the flap till it comes out from the other end. Then move the dissector outwards so that the flap is created (Fig. 6.2). The flap is then lifted and any bleeding vessel can be cauterized.

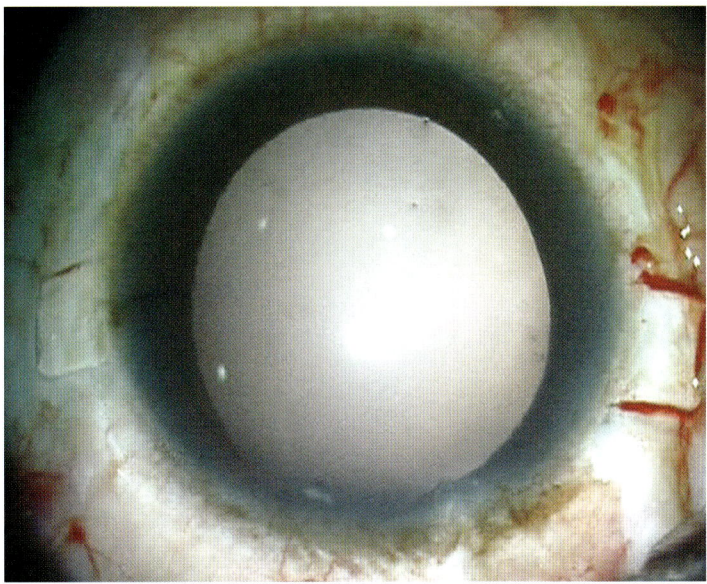

Fig. 6.2 Two partial scleral thickness flaps made 180 degrees opposite to each other

Infusion with a Trocar Cannula

One should get infusion of fluid into the eye. This can be done using a sutureless 23 G/25 G trocar cannula (Fig. 6.3). The advantage is that there is no disruption of conjunctival integrity, no need for suturing the sclerotomy, and a reduction in surgical time. Insertion and removal of the cannula is faster than with a conventional 20-gauge infusion cannula. The trocar infusion kit is available separately and can be used by anterior segment surgeons in special situations. It contains a scleral guide, an inserter, and an infusion cannula. The scleral guide is inserted into the pars plana about 3.0 mm from the limbus with the help of the inserter, the inserter is removed, and the infusion cannula connected to the infusion bottle is then inserted. During removal of the cannula, the infusion is switched off and the scleral guide removed. No suture is applied in the sclerotomy site. We noted that the surgical time needed to fixate the infusion cannula was reduced when 23-gauge infusion was used. It was also safe and easy in the hands of the anterior segment surgeons as one had to insert only the trocar and fixate the infusion cannula. One should always ensure the tip of the infusion cannula is in the vitreous cavity before the infusion is started. If the pupil is miotic, an iris retractor can be used to retract the iris and check that the infusion cannula is in the vitreous cavity. The direct visualization of the cannula during entrance and exit decreases the risk for complications.

Fixating a normal 20-gauge infusion cannula requires time to cut the conjunctiva, perform cautery, and then suture the infusion cannula to the sclera. Compared with the 20-gauge infusion cannula, the 23-gauge cannula caused

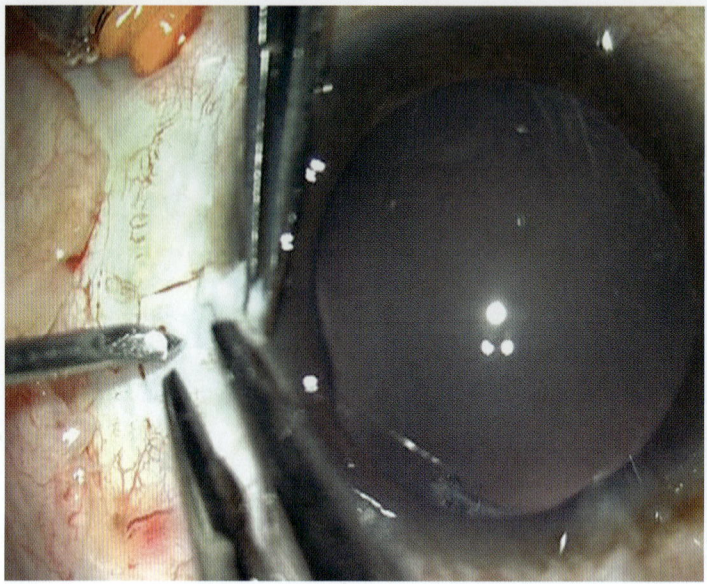

Fig. 6.3 Infusion introduced into the eye with trocar-cannula. Sclerotomy is being done with a 20 G needle approximately 1 mm from the limbus, beneath the scleral flaps

significantly less postoperative pain and discomfort. In summary, if a 23-gauge trocar cannula kit is readily available in the operating room, it would be easy to use in glued IOL implantation by the anterior segment surgeon.

Infusion with an Anterior Chamber Maintainer

Another alternative is to fix an anterior chamber (AC) maintainer in the eye. For this one has to make a clear corneal incision with a side port knife and then pass the AC maintainer in the eye. It should be parallel to the iris and in an area which does not affect the surgical view.

Trocar Cannula vs Anterior Chamber Maintainer

Infusion of fluid can be done with either a trocar cannula or an AC maintainer. The advantage of a trocar cannula is that as it is in the vitreous cavity it does not hamper the surgical view. It also does not push back the iris or touch the iris. The disadvantage is that an anterior segment surgeon might not have easy access to a trocar cannula compared to a posterior segment surgeon. Another problem is that one should check the trocar cannula is in the vitreous cavity before turning on the infusion so that the fluid does not go into the subretinal space. Sometimes this may be difficult to visualize in small pupils, etc.

The advantage of an AC maintainer is that it is easily available, is re-autoclavable and also there is no issue of one having to be careful that the tip is in the subretinal space. The disadvantage of an AC maintainer is that the clear corneal incision does not always match the size of the AC maintainer accurately. This can lead to extrusion of the AC maintainer from the corneal incision in the middle of surgery and would then have to be refixed. Another issue with the AC maintainer is that when the fluid is turned on it pushes the iris back creating a deep anterior chamber. When one has to make the 20-gauge needle sclerotomy under the scleral flaps one can hit the iris root as the iris is pushed back by the fluid. A solution to this problem is to fix the AC maintainer, create the 20-gauge sclerotomies and then turn on the infusion.

Scleral Flaps or Infusion—Which Comes First?

One has to decide whether to create the scleral flaps first or fix the infusion for fluid. If one is operating a fresh case for example a patient posted for secondary IOL in aphakia or a fresh ectopia lentis, it is better to create the scleral flaps first. The reason is that the globe is firm and it is easy to create the scleral flaps. In a case of a posterior capsular rupture where the corneal or scleral tunnel is open and one is preparing for a glued IOL surgery, it is better to first fix the infusion. This way fluid is flowing inside the eye. One can suture the open wound (either clear corneal or scleral tunnel) then fix the infusion for fluid. This way the globe becomes firm and it is easy to create the scleral flaps. Creating the scleral flaps in eyes which are open is tricky as the eye ball is soft.

Sclerotomies Under the Flap

Two straight sclerotomies with a 20 G needle are made about 1.0 mm from the limbus under the existing scleral flaps (Fig. 6.3). The sclerotomies are to be directed obliquely into the mid-vitreous cavity so that it does not hit the iris which can happen if the sclerotomies are made in a horizontal direction. If one is using a 23-gauge glued IOL forceps one can make a 20-gauge sclerotomy. If one is using a 22-gauge needle for the sclerotomy then one has to use a 25-gauge glued IOL forceps for externalizing the haptics.

Vitrectomy

Vitrectomy is performed using a 20/23/25 G vitrectomy probe (Fig. 6.4). A good vitrectomy is crucial so that there is no vitreous traction and chances of retinal breaks and retinal detachments are nullified. If one is using a 23/25 G vitrectomy probe which are available with posterior vitrectomy machines one can pass the probe through the sclerotomy under the scleral flap. If one is using the vitrectomy set up of a phaco machine one should remember that those vitrectomy probes are 20 G and will not pass through the 20 G needle sclerotomies. In such a case one should make a clear corneal incision and do the vitrectomy through the clear corneal incision.

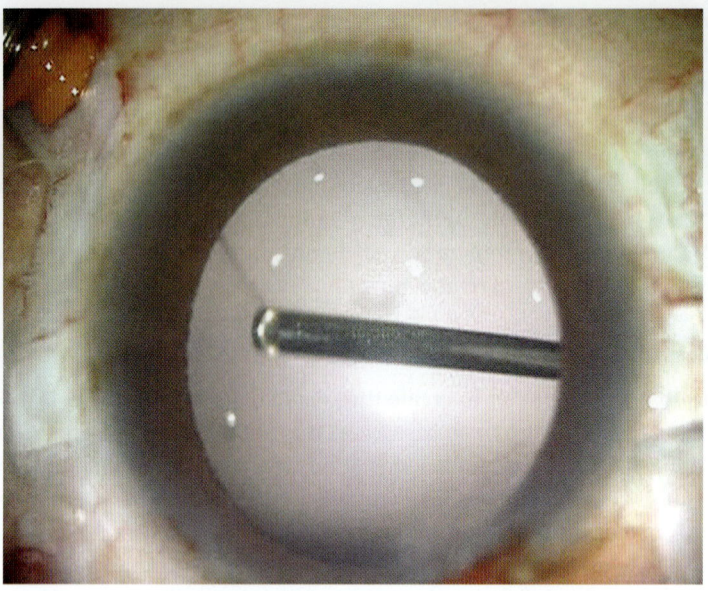

Fig. 6.4 23 G vitrectomy probe introduced from the sclerotomy site. Vitrectomy is being done to clear vitreous in the pupillary plane and anterior chamber

Intraocular Lens Types

Glued IOL can be performed well with rigid polymethylmethacrylate (PMMA) IOL, 3-piece PCIOL or IOLs with modified PMMA haptics. Therefore one does not need to have an entire inventory of special sutured scleral fixated SFIOLs with eyelets. In dislocated PC PMMA IOL or three piece IOLs, the same IOL can be repositioned thereby reducing the need for further manipulation. The IOL that cannot be glued is the single piece foldable IOL as one needs a firm haptic to tuck and glue.

The best IOL to use is a 3-piece IOL as the haptics do not break compared to a single piece nonfoldable IOL. A foldable 3-piece IOL is even better for a simple reason that the incision has not to be enlarged. The length of a normal foldable 3-piece IOL is 13 mm. The Staar® surgical lens is 13.5 mm which makes it better for glued IOL surgery as one will have more haptic externalized. The 3-piece non foldable IOL's are also 13.5 mm.

Foldable Intraocular Lens Injectors

It is preferable to have a plunger-type injector for better coordination although a screwing mechanism type injector may also be used. In the latter case, the assistant gently maneuvers the IOL forward as the surgeon holds the injector with one hand and the glued IOL forceps with the other hand. While introducing the injector, it is advisable to have the injector tip within the mouth of the incision and not use wound-assisted injection of the IOL that can lead to a sudden, uncontrolled entry of the IOL into the eye and a consequent IOL drop into the vitreous.

Leading Haptic Externalization

When we are using a foldable IOL one has to take a 3-piece foldable IOL. Once the lens is loaded to see that the haptic is slightly out of the cartridge. The cartridge is introduced into the AC. The glued IOL forceps is passed through the sclerotomy and it grasps the tip of the haptic (Fig. 6.5). The IOL is then gradually injected into the eye. If the injector is a screwing mechanism one then the assistant screws the injector. One should not externalize the haptic till the optic totally unfolds inside the eye, otherwise the optic can break. Once the optic has unfolded (Fig. 6.6), the glued IOL forceps pulls the haptic out and externalizes it. The haptic can then be caught by an assistant (Fig. 6.7).

At this stage, George Beiko from Canada has suggested to put the silicone plugs of an iris hook onto the haptic which has been externalized to prevent the haptic from slipping back. Priya Narang from India has suggested a no-assistant technique where the trailing haptic is passed into the eye near the inferior portion so that due to the principles of vector forces the leading haptic cannot slip back.

When one is injecting the IOL, one hand is holding the tip of the haptic. Fear of the IOL falling into the vitreous cavity is not there as:

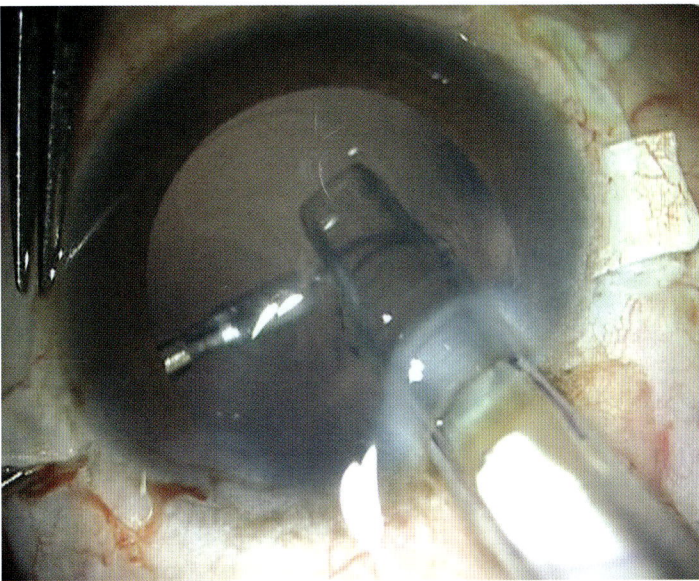

Fig. 6.5 A 3-piece foldable IOL is loaded and being unfolded in the eye. The tip of the leading haptic is grasped with MST forceps (Glued IOL forceps)

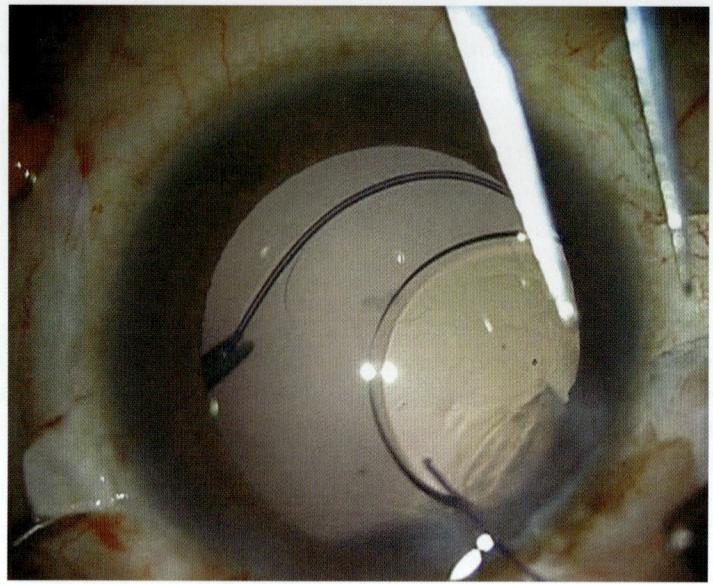

Fig. 6.6 The surgeon waits for the entire IOL to unfold

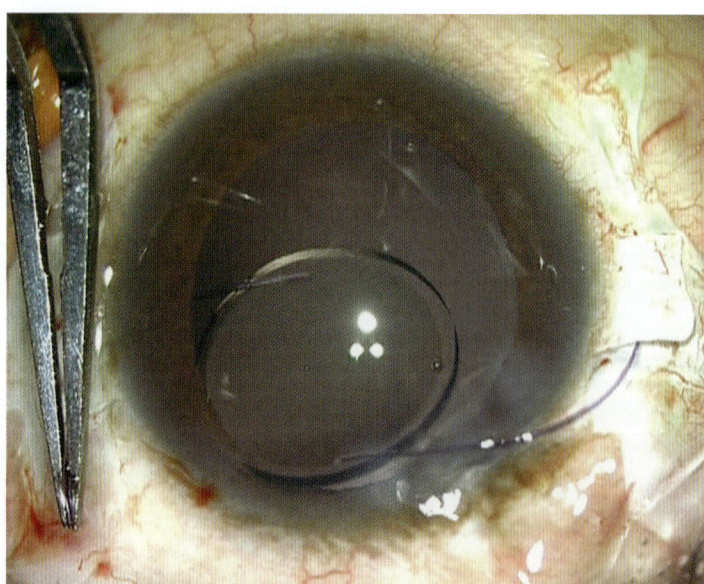

Fig. 6.7 The leading haptic is externalized and grasped by an assistant to prevent its slippage into the eye

- The tip of the haptic is caught with the forceps so the IOL cannot go down
- The trailing haptic is still outside the eye. If the forceps slips and the haptic is missed the trailing haptic can still be caught and the IOL would not fall into the vitreous cavity.

Trailing Haptic Externalization

The trailing haptic is caught with the glued IOL forceps and flexed into the AC (Fig. 6.8). The haptic is transferred from the first forceps to the second using the handshake technique. The second forceps is passed through the side port. The first forceps is then passed through the sclerotomy under the scleral flap. The haptic is transferred from the second forceps back to the first using the hand shake technique once again (Fig. 6.9). The haptic tip is grasped with the first forceps and pulled towards the sclerotomy and externalized.

Vitrectomy Around the Sclerotomy

While all these maneuvers are being done some vitreous might be in the sclerotomy site. Vitrectomy should be done around the sclerotomy (Fig. 6.10). Then one should asses the IOL position. Without anyone holding the IOL, the lens must be stable. If the haptic is slipping back then it is possible:
- The eye is large and has a large WTW in which case a vertical glued IOL would have to be done

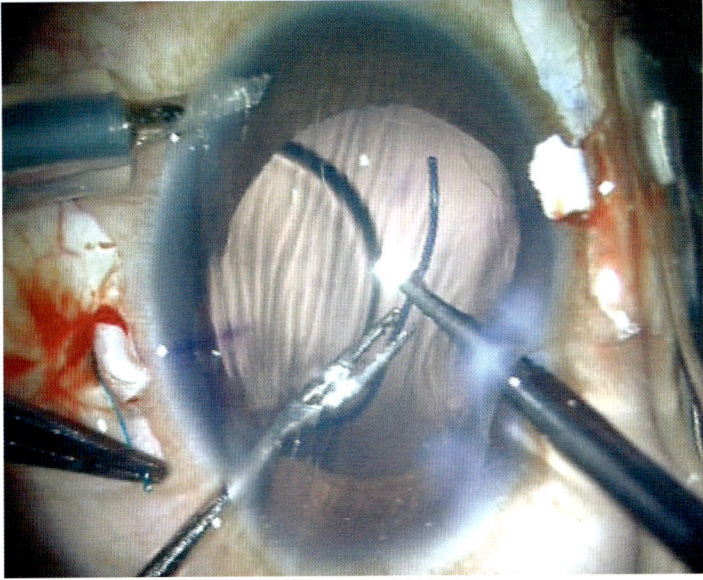

Fig. 6.8 The trailing haptic is flexed in the eye and an MST forceps is introduced from the side port incision. The trailing haptic is then grasped by left hand

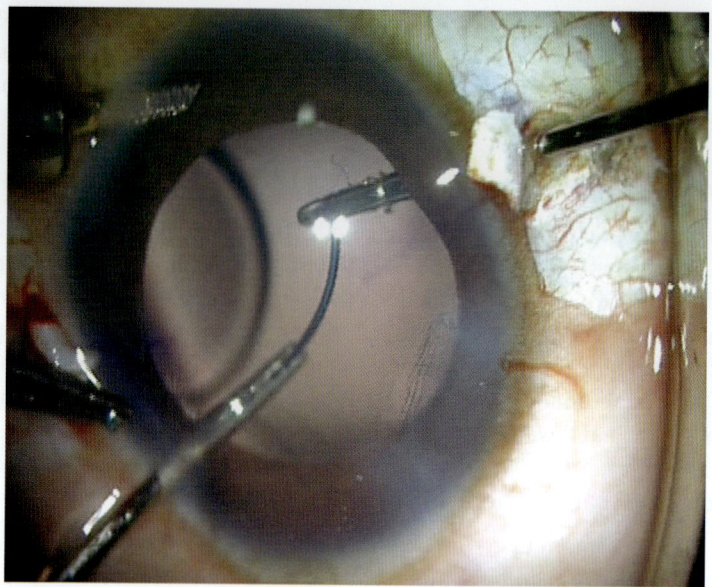

Fig. 6.9 The surgeon withdraws the right hand and re-introduces the MST forceps from the right sclerotomy site. The haptic is then transferred from left to right hand

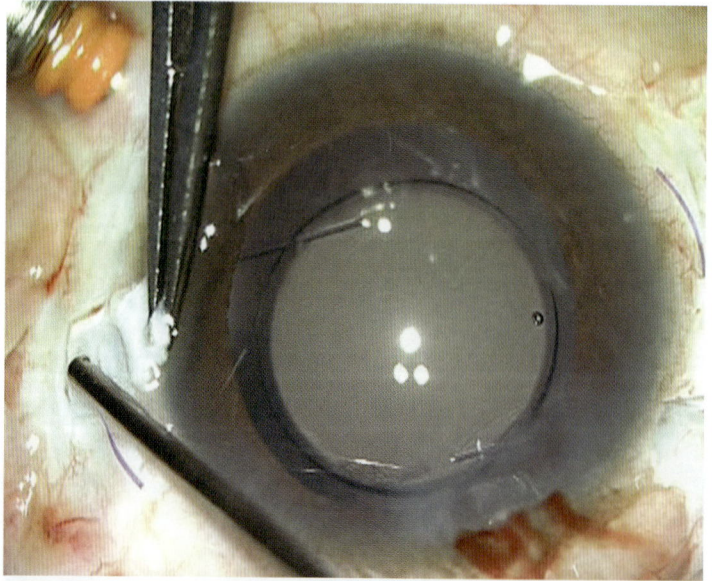

Fig. 6.10 Vitrectomy is done at sclerotomy site to cut down all vitreous strands

- The sclerotomy made is too far back so very little haptic has been externalized.

If the haptics are slipping back then a fresh sclerotomy should be made more anterior to the previous one, the haptic pushed back into the vitreous cavity and using the handshake technique again grasped and re-externalized through the fresh anterior sclerotomy. Once again assessment should be made if the IOL is stable without tucking and gluing.

Scharioth Scleral Pocket and Intrascleral Haptic Tuck

Gabor Scharioth from Germany started the first intrascleral haptic fixation in 2006. It is the intrascleral haptic fixation which gives stability to the IOL. A 26-gauge needle is taken and bent so that it is like a keratome. The 26-gauge needle then creates a scleral tunnel at the edge of the flap where the haptic is externalized. The haptic is then flexed and tucked into the scleral pocket (Figs 6.11 to 6.13). One can also mark the Scharioth scleral pocket and create it even before the eye is opened. The 26-gauge needle is marked with the marker pen to leave a mark in the sclera where the scleral pocket is created. This can be done adjacent to the area where the sclerotomy will be made. It is now easy to know where the scleral pocket is located. Another way is to pass a rod in the area of the scleral pocket to check its location.

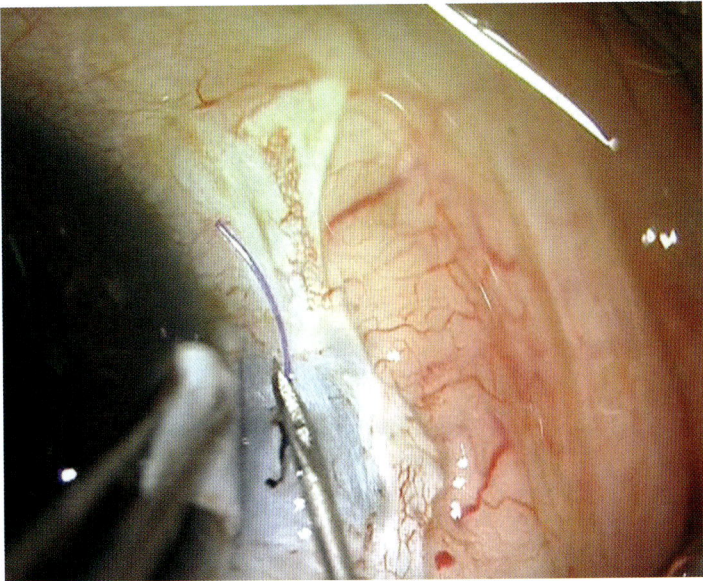

Fig. 6.11 Site for scleral pocket chosen. It should be parallel to the sclerotomy site and along the edge of the scleral flap wall

Management of PHACO Complications: Newer Techniques

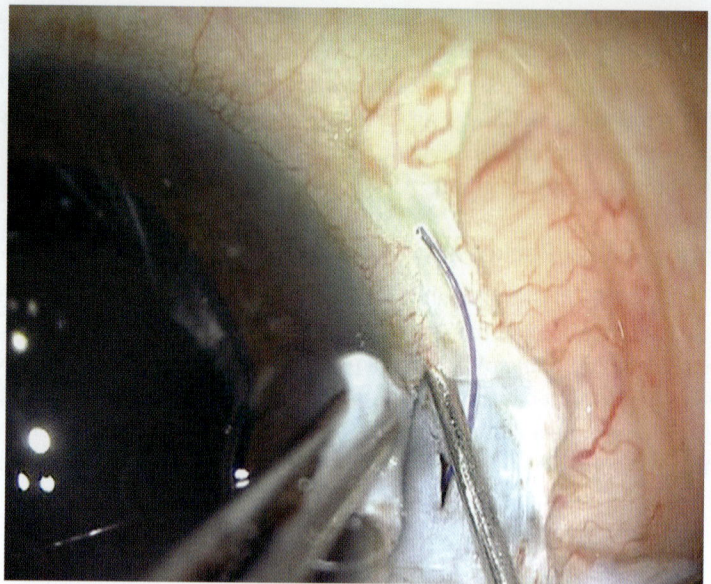

Fig. 6.12 Scleral pocket is made with a 26 G needle

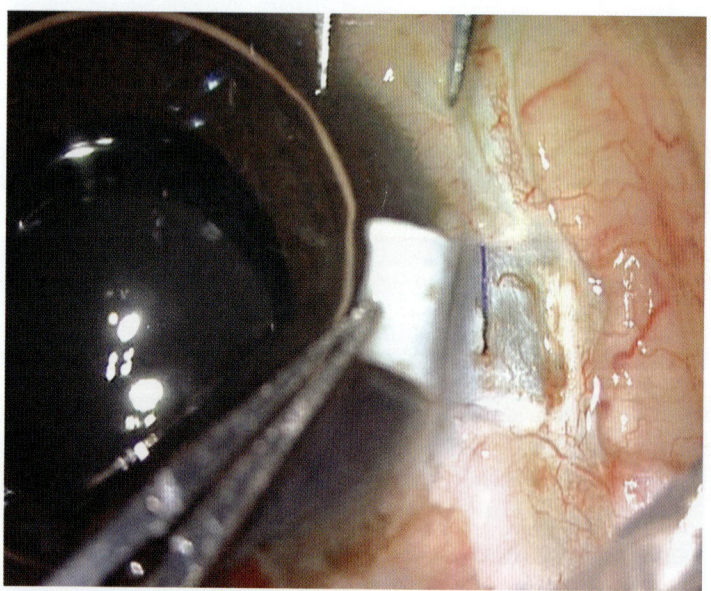

Fig. 6.13 Haptic tucked in scleral pocket

Air in the Anterior Chamber

Air is now injected into the AC and the fluid from the infusion cannula is turned off. The fibrin glue has to work in a dry area so the fluid has to be turned off. Otherwise fluid might keep on coming from the sclerotomy site. Once fluid is turned off, there could be intraoperative hypotony and also postoperative hypotony. To prevent this, we inject air in the AC to have a firm globe intra-and postoperatively (Fig. 6.14).

Fibrin Glue

The fibrin kit we use is Reliseal (Reliance Life Sciences, India) or TISSEEL (Baxter, USA). The fibrinogen and thrombin are first reconstituted according to the manufacturer's instructions. The commercially available fibrin glue (FG) is virus inactivated and is checked for viral antigen and antibodies with polymerase chain reaction; hence, the chances of transmission of infection are very low. The glue is applied beneath the flaps (Fig. 6.14) and after sealing them. It can be used over the conjunctiva and clear corneal incisions to seal them too.

Role of Fibrin Glue

The fibrin glue plays a multifactorial role in glued IOL surgery.
- The glue helps seal the haptic to the sclera which gives extra support to the intrascleral haptic tuck.

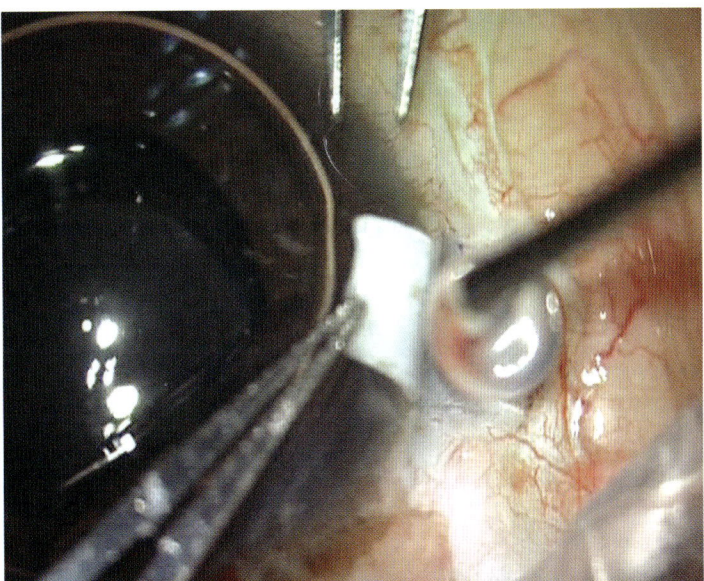

Fig. 6.14 Fibrin glue applied beneath the scleral flaps for adhesion

- The glue seals the flaps so that there is no opening from inside the eye to the outside. This prevents any chances of endophthalmitis even some years later where one could get conjunctivitis leading to endophthalmitis as there is an opening from inside to the outside of the eye.
- The glue prevents any trabeculectomy opening as the flaps are now firmly stuck.
- The glue helps seal the cut conjunctiva.
- The glue helps seal the clear corneal incisions.

Postoperative Regimen

One should keep a watch on the patients postoperatively as these are worst case scenarios being operated upon. They need postoperative antibiotic steroids for 6 weeks. If there is a temporary elevation of IOP, antiglaucoma medications can be given. If there is a reaction then subconjunctival antibiotic-steroids can also be given.

Stability of the Intraocular Lens Haptic

As the flaps are manually created, the rough opposing surfaces of the flap and bed heal rapidly and firmly around the haptic, being helped by the fibrin glue early on. The major uncertainty here is the stability of the fibrin matrix *in vivo*. Numerous animal studies have shown that the fibrin glue is still present at 4 to 6 weeks. Because postoperative fibrosis starts early, the flaps become stuck secondary to fibrosis even prior to full degradation of the glue. The ensuing fibrosis acts as a firm scaffold around the haptic which prevents movement along the long axis (Fig. 6.15). To further make the IOL rock stable, we tuck the haptic tip into the scleral wall through a tunnel. This prevents all movement of the haptic along the transverse axis as well (Fig. 6.16). The stability of the lens first comes through the tucking of the haptics in the scleral pocket created. The tissue glue then gives it extra stability and also seals the flap down. Externalization of the greater part of the haptics along its curvature stabilizes the axial positioning of the IOL and thereby prevents any IOL tilt.

Advantages

This fibrin glue assisted sutureless PCIOL implantation technique would be useful in a myriad of clinical situations where scleral fixated IOLs are indicated, such as, luxated IOL, dislocated IOL, zonulopathy or secondary IOL implantation.

No special intraocular lenses needed: It can be performed well with rigid PMMA IOL, 3-piece PCIOL or IOLs with modified PMMA haptics. In dislocated posterior chamber PMMA IOL, the same IOL can be repositioned thereby reducing the need for further manipulation.

Glued Intrascleral Haptic Fixation of Intraocular Lens (Glued IOL)

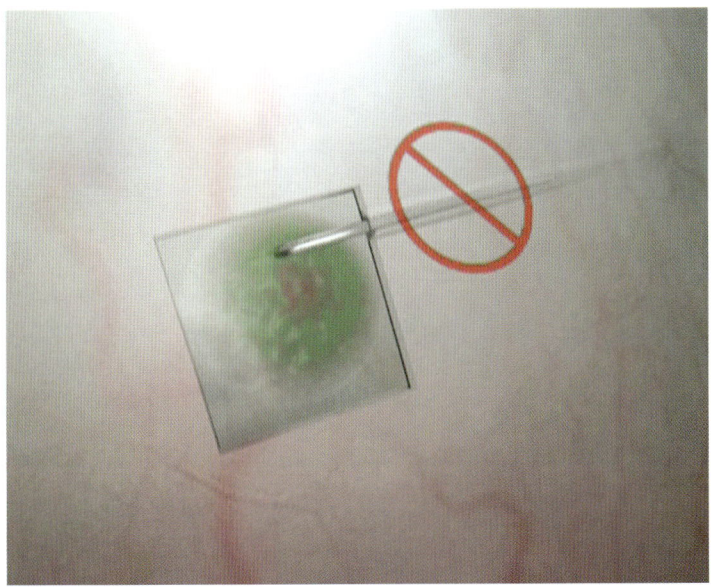

Fig. 6.15 Any longitudinal movement of the haptic is avoided due to tucking

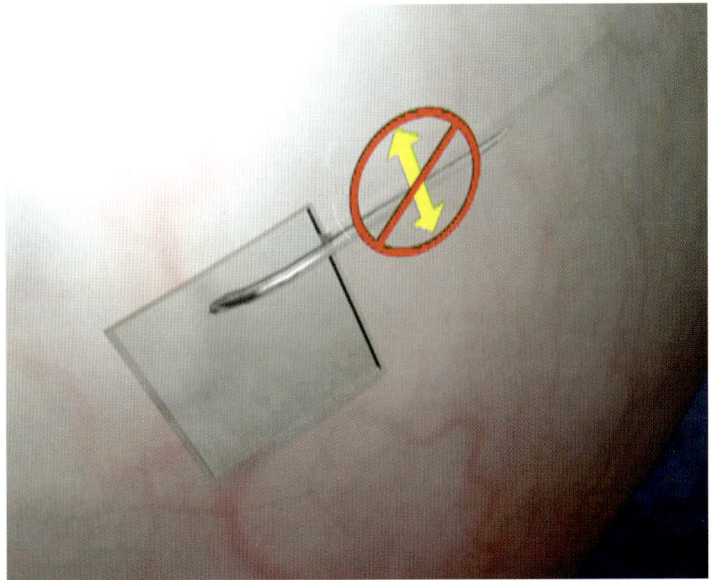

Fig. 6.16 Horizontal movement of the haptic is nullified by tucking

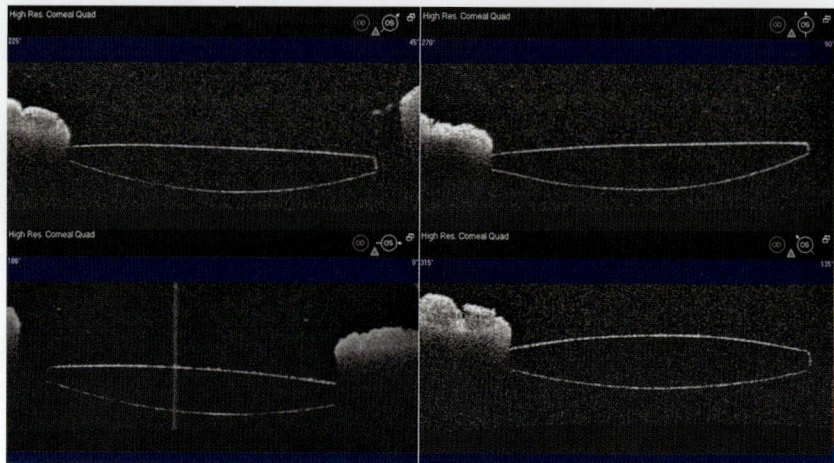

Fig. 6.17 Ocular coherence tomography (OCT) shows no optic tilt

No tilt: Since the overall diameter of the routine IOL is about 12 to 13 mm, with the haptic being placed in its normal curved configuration and without any traction, there is no distortion or change in shape of the IOL optic (Fig. 6.17). Externalization of the greater part of the haptics along its curvature stabilizes the axial positioning of the IOL and thereby prevents any IOL tilt.

Less pseudophacodonesis: When the eye moves, it acquires kinetic energy from its muscles and attachments and the energy is dissipated to the internal fluids as it stops. Thus pseudophacodonesis is the result of oscillations of the fluids in the anterior and posterior segment of the eye. These oscillations, initiated by movement of the eye, result in shearing forces on the corneal endothelium as well as vitreous motion lead to permanent damage. Since the IOL haptic is stuck beneath the flap, it would prevent the further movement of the haptic and thereby reducing the pseudophacodonesis.

Less uveitis-glaucoma-hyphema (UGH) syndrome: We expect less incidence of UGH syndrome in fibrin glue assisted IOL implantation as compared to sutured scleral fixated IOL. This is because, in the former the IOL is well-stabilized and stuck onto the scleral bed and thereby, has decreased intraocular mobility whereas in the latter, there is increased possibility of IOL movement or persistent rub over the ciliary body.

No suture related complications: Visually significant complications due to late subluxation which has been known to occur in sutured scleral fixated IOL may also be prevented as sutures are totally avoided in this technique. Another important advantage of this technique is the prevention of suture related complications like suture erosion, suture knot exposure or dislocation of IOL after suture disintegration or broken suture.

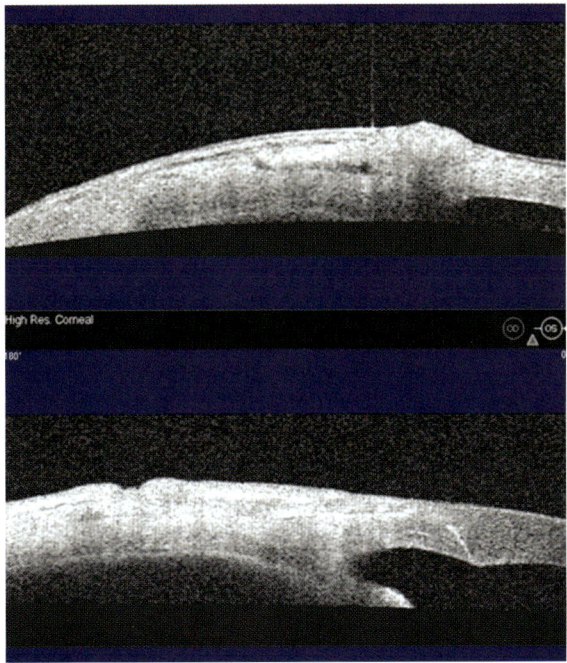

Fig. 6.18 Well-adhered scleral flaps are seen on anterior segment ocular coherence tomography (OCT)

Rapidity and ease of surgery: Since all the time taken in SFIOL for passing suture into the IOL haptic eyelets, to ensure good centration before tying down the knots as well as time for suturing scleral flaps and closing conjunctiva are significantly reduced. The risk of retinal photic injury which is known to occur in SFIOL would also be reduced in our technique due to the short surgical time. Fibrin glue takes less time [Reliseal (20 seconds)/TISSEEL (3 secs)] to act in the scleral bed and it helps in adhesion as well as hemostasis. The preparation time can also be reduced in elective procedures by preparing it prior to surgery as it remains stable up to 4 hours from the time of reconstitution. Fibrin glue has been shown to provide airtight closure and by the time the fibrin starts degrading, surgical adhesions would have already occurred in the scleral bed. This is well-shown in the follow-up anterior segment OCT (Fig. 6.18) where postoperative perfect scleral flap adhesion is observed.

REFERENCES

1. Vajpayee RB, Sharma N, Dada T, et al. Management of posterior capsule tears. Surv Ophthal. 2001;45:473-88.
2. Wu MC, Bhandari A. Managing the broken capsule. Curr Opin Ophthalmol. 2008;19:36-40.

3. Agarwal A, Kumar DA, Jacob S, et al. Fibrin glue–assisted sutureless posterior chamber intraocular lens implantation in eyes with deficient posterior capsules. J Cataract Refract Surg. 2008;34:1433-8.
4. Prakash G, Kumar DA, Jacob S, et al. Anterior segment optical coherence tomography-aided diagnosis and primary posterior chamber intraocular lens implantation with fibrin glue in traumatic phacocele with scleral perforation. J Cataract Refract Surg. 2009;35:782-4.
5. Prakash G, Jacob S, Kumar DA, et al. Femtosecond assisted keratoplasty with fibrin glue–assisted sutureless posterior chamber lens implantation: a new triple procedure. J Cataract Refract Surg. In press (manuscript no. 08-919).
6. Agarwal A, Kumar DA, Prakash G, et al. Fibrin glue–assisted sutureless posterior chamber intraocular lens implantation in eyes with deficient posterior capsules [Reply to letter]. J Cataract Refract Surg. 2009;35:795-6.
7. Nair V, Kumar DA, Prakash G, et al. Bilateral spontaneous in-the-bag anterior subluxation of PCIOL managed with glued IOL technique: A case report, Eye Contact Lens 2009. In Press (manuscript no. ECL-07-281).
8. Gabor SGB, Pavilidis MM. Sutureless intrascleral posterior chamber intraocular lens fixation. J Cataract Refract Surg. 2007;33:1851-4.
9. Maggi R, Maggi C. Sutureless scleral fixation of intraocular lenses. J Cataract Refract Surg. 1997;23:1289-94.
10. Teichmann KD, Teichmann IAM. The torque and tilt gamble. J Cataract Refract Surg. 1997;23:413-8.
11. Jacobi KW, Jagger WS. Physical forces involved in pseudophacodonesis and iridodonesis. Albrecht Von Graefes Arch Klin Exp Ophthalmol. 1981;216:49-53.
12. Price MO, Price FW Jr, Werner L, et al. Late dislocation of scleral-sutured posterior chamber intraocular lenses. J Cataract Refract Surg. 2005;31(7):1320-6.
13. Solomon K, Gussler JR, Gussler C, Van Meter WS. Incidence and management of complications of transsclerally sutured posterior chamber lenses. J Cataract Refract Surg. 1993;19:488-93.
14. Asadi R, Kheirkhah A. Long-term results of scleral fixation of posterior chamber intraocular lenses in children. Ophthalmology. 2008;115(1):67-72. Epub 2007 May 3.
15. Lanzetta P, Menchini U, Virgili G, et al. Scleral fixated intraocular lenses: an angiographic study. Retina. 1998;18:515-20.

CHAPTER **7**

Handshake Technique for Glued IOL

Priya Narang, Amar Agarwal

INTRODUCTION

Glued IOL as a technique for PCIOL fixation in eyes with absent or insufficient capsular support was first described by us in 2007.[1-9] Since then a large number of cases have been done with this technique. The technique has evolved since then and extended its application to many different scenarios and as a part of combined surgeries.[4,7,8] 'Handshake' technique is a modification in the glued IOL procedure in which the IOL haptic is bimanually transferred from one end opening forceps to another under direct visualization in the pupillary plane.

LEADING HAPTIC EXTERNALIZATION

One of the greatest changes was the use of foldable IOLs for performing this surgery thus extending all the advantages that a small incision offers. Any three piece foldable IOL can be used for this technique. Depending on surgeon preference, an infusion cannula or AC maintainer is fixed and the flaps and sclerotomies made. A 2.8 mm keratome is used to make a corneal incision. This may be enlarged very slightly so as to allow easy insertion. A side port may also be made to allow the surgeon easier maneuverability and as a future access point if required. The three piece foldable IOL is loaded into the injector. The extreme tip of the haptic is left protruding out to allow the MST forceps to grab it easily. The injector tip is then introduced into the AC (Figs 7.1A to E). At the same time, a 23 G glued IOL (Microsurgical technology, MST, USA) forceps is then introduced through the sclerotomy under the scleral flap. As the IOL is being injected into the AC, the tip of the haptic is caught with the MST forceps and exteriorized while injection is continued very gently. The injector is then slowly withdrawn so that the second haptic is left trailing outside the wound. The first haptic is then held by an assistant.

TRAILING HAPTIC EXTERNALIZATION

The surgeon now flexes the second haptic into the AC into the jaws of an MST forceps introduced through the second sclerotomy. This haptic is also thus

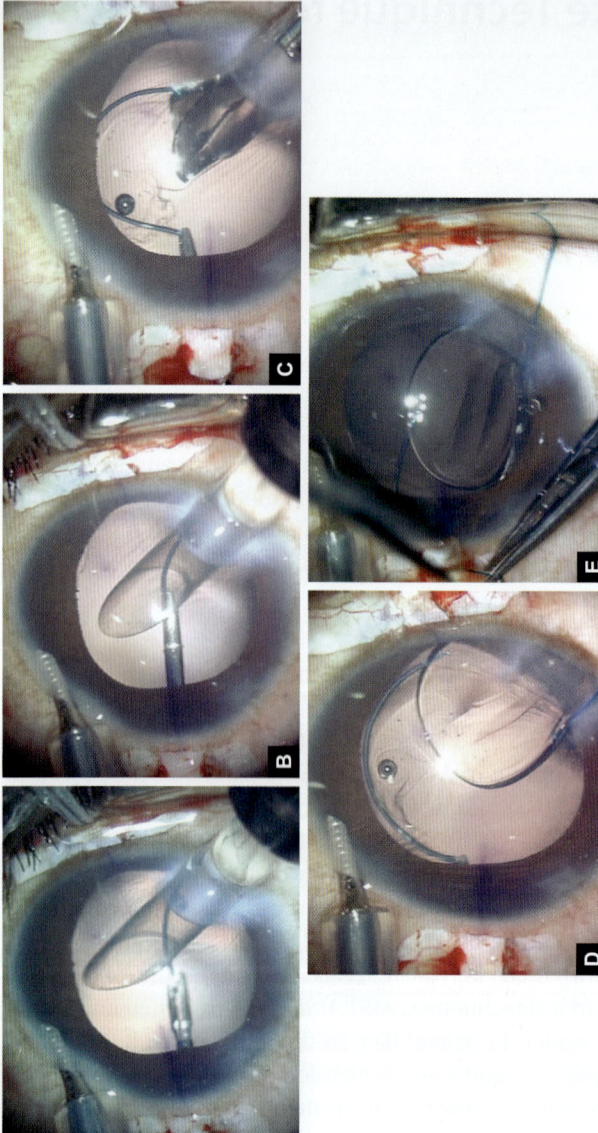

Figs 7.1A to E Leading haptic externalization in glued IOL. (A) IOL in injector. Note the haptic tip is slightly out of the cartridge. Also cartridge is in the AC. There is no wound assisted injection. Glued IOL forceps (Epsilon, India) is passed through the sclerotomy with the other hand ready to grasp the tip of the haptic. One should not do wound assisted as the injection might happen too fast. This can either break the IOL or push it so fast it might go into the vitreous cavity; (B) Tip of the haptic grasped with the glued IOL forceps; (C) Injection of the IOL continued, if it is a plunger type injector surgeon can do it, but if it is a screwing mechanism injector, assistant can screw the injector for release of the IOL as both hands of the surgeon are occupied; (D) IOL has unfolded inside the eye, then only cartridge is removed. Note one hand still holding the haptic tip but not yet externalized the tip. If one externalizes the haptic before the IOL has unfolded from the cartridge the IOL can break; (E) Haptic externalized and assistant tries to grasp the haptic so that haptic does not fall back inside the eye

externalized out (Figs 7.2A to F). In a routine foldable glued IOL, the MST forceps can also be introduced through the side port to grasp the trailing forceps and feed it into the jaws of the second MST forceps. Depending on ease of access, the other MST forceps is introduced through the opposite sclerotomy or through the side-port.

SCHARIOTH TUCK AND GLUE

A bent 26 gauge needle is then used to create a tunnel in the direction of the exteriorized haptics at the edge of the scleral flap. Vitrectomy is then used to clear up the scleral bed in case any vitreous has prolapsed out. Both haptics are then tucked intrasclerally. Centration of the IOL is checked for and if not well centered, the degree of tuck of the individual haptics is adjusted till the lens becomes well centered. The scleral bed is then dried, fibrin glue applied and the scleral flaps are glued down. Fibrin glue is also used to seal the mainport and the sideport corneal incisions by applying glue over the incisions. The conjunctiva is also closed with fibrin glue.

INJECTOR

It is preferable to have a plunger type injector for better coordination though a screw mechanism type injector may also be used. In the latter case, the assistant gently maneuvers the IOL forwards as the surgeon holds the injector with one hand and the MST forceps with the other hand. While introducing the injector, it is advisable to have the injector tip within the mouth of the incision and not use wound assisted injection of the IOL which can lead to a sudden, uncontrolled entry of the IOL into the eye and a consequent IOL drop into the vitreous.

HANDSHAKE TECHNIQUE FOR FOLDABLE GLUED IOL

We have seen that exteriorization of the haptics is a key step in performing glued IOL. Since the surgeon is maneuvering with both hands simultaneously, one hand injecting the IOL while the other grasps and exteriorizes the haptics, he/she needs to be familiar with the handshake technique as a means of transferring the haptic from one hand to the other. The handshake technique can be utilized in a variety of situations. For example, it is essential to hold the haptic at its tip before exteriorizing it so that it does not snag on the sclerotomy while being brought out. The handshake transfer of the haptic between the two MST forceps is continued till the tip of the haptic is caught by the forceps on the side to which the haptic is to be exteriorized. Another situation is if one of the haptics is not caught or if it gets released accidentally after grasping it. In this case too, the handshake technique can be used to regrasp the haptic. The MST forceps is introduced through the side port which becomes invaluable in this situation. The handshake technique utilizes two MST forceps, one of which holds one haptic (Figs 7.3A to F). The other

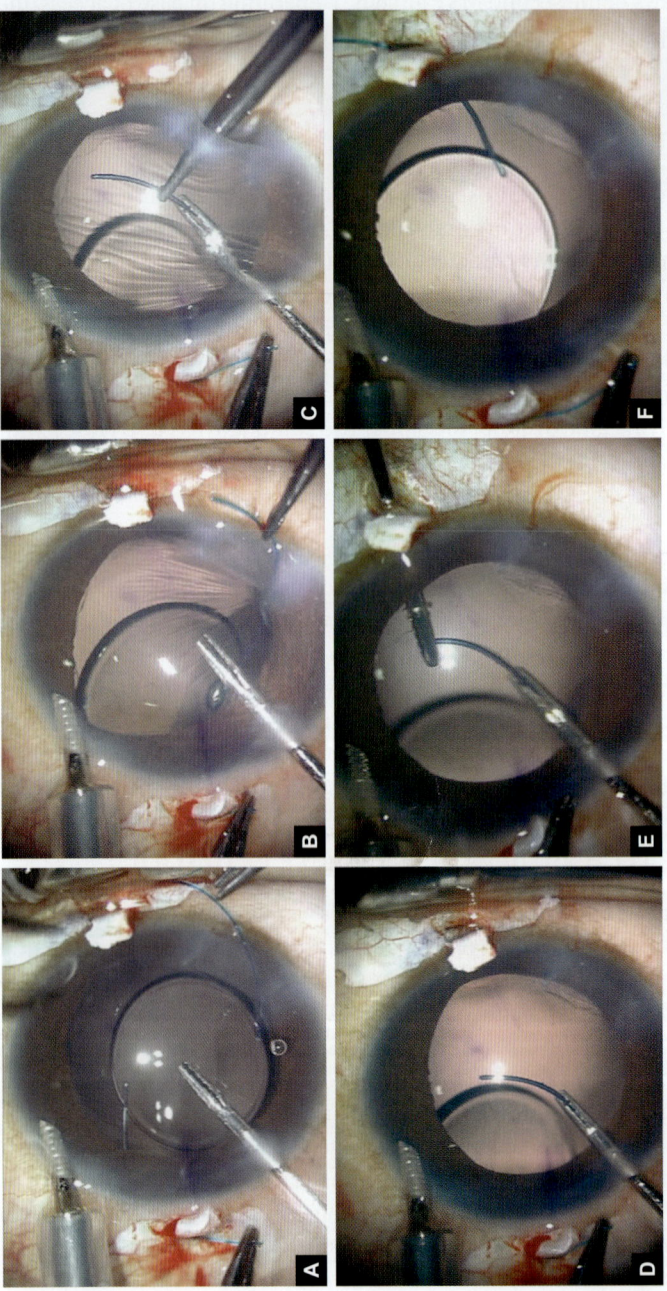

Figs 7.2A to F Handshake technique for trailing haptic. (A) Glued IOL forceps (Epsilon, India) passed through the side port; (B) The trailing haptic grasped with a forceps and flexed to make it enter the AC; (C) Trailing haptic passed into the AC and with handshake technique, haptic grasp shifted from one forceps to the other. Note the dimpling on the cornea as the main incision is open due to the forceps passage; (D) Trailing haptic caught with forceps passed through the side port. Note no dimpling on the cornea as main port incision is closed. It is now easy to see the tip of the haptic; (E) Glued IOL forceps passed through the sclerotomy and tip of the haptic grasped. Once again handshake technique helps pass the haptic from one forceps to the other; (F) Trailing haptic externalized

Handshake Technique for Glued IOL

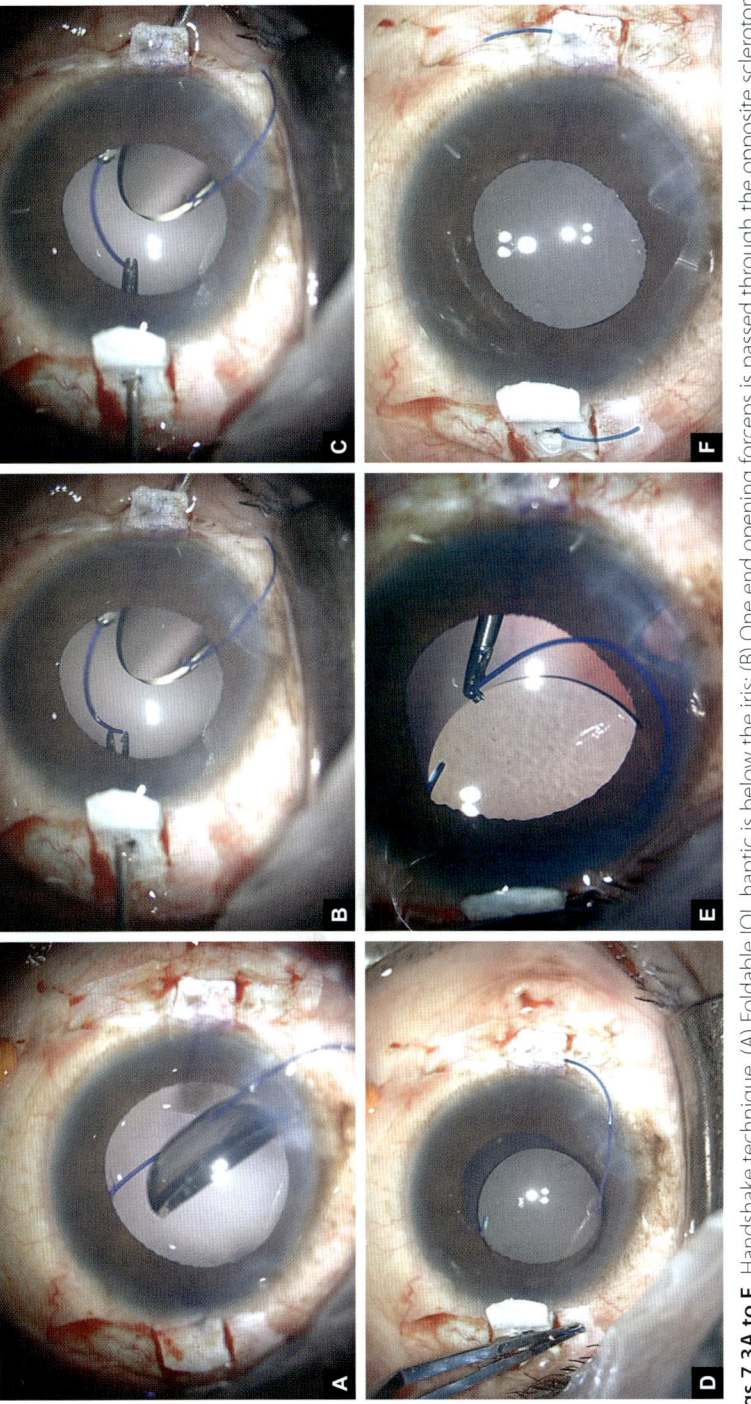

Figs 7.3A to F Handshake technique. (A) Foldable IOL haptic is below the iris; (B) One end opening forceps is passed through the opposite sclerotomy site while other forceps is ready to receive the haptic; (C) The leading haptic is grasped with forceps and the haptic tip is fed into another forceps; (D) One haptic externalized and assistant holds the haptic; (E) Trailing haptic caught with the end opening forceps; (F) Both the haptics externalized under the scleral flaps

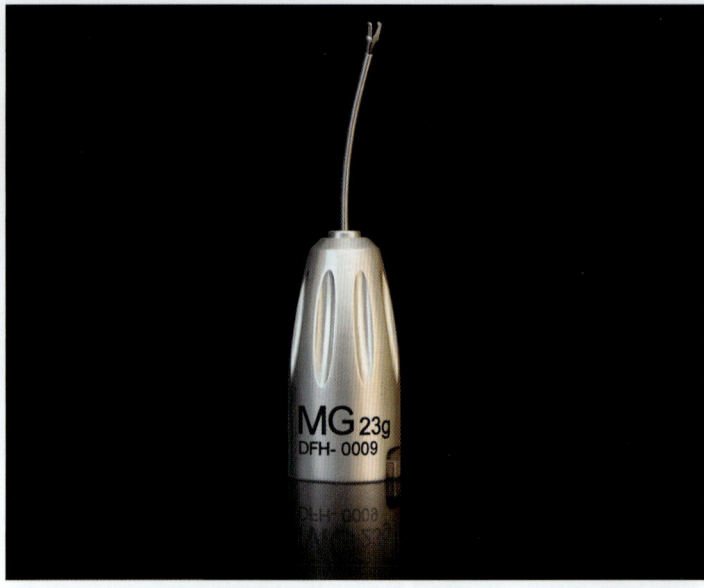

Fig. 7.4 Ahmed micrograsper. End opening forceps for glued IOL surgery—(Microsurgical technology MST, USA) (*Courtesy:* Larry Laks, MST, USA)

MST forceps is then introduced into the eye and the first hand then transfers the haptic into the second MST forceps such that the first hand now becomes free. This technique is especially useful in subluxated three piece IOLs as it allows easy intraocular maneuverability of the entire haptic or IOL within a closed globe system. The MST forceps is introduced through the sclerotomy to grasp the IOL while vitrectomy is done all around the IOL to free vitreous traction. Once the IOL is free, an MST forceps (Fig. 7.4) is introduced through the other sclerotomy site and the IOL is exchanged between hands till the tip of the haptic is grasped. This haptic is then exteriorized and held by the assistant while the handshake maneuver is used for the second haptic in a similar manner. This allows refixation of the same IOL with a closed chamber approach with minimal intervention.

CONCLUSION

The foldable glued IOL technique and the handshake technique further refine this procedure by the use of smaller incisions and better intraocular maneuverability, making it possible to perform the entire procedure through small self sealing incisions. This has the intraoperative advantages of having a well formed globe throughout all the steps of surgery. It eliminates iris prolapse during IOL insertion and wound suturing and also significantly decreases time of surgery as there is no need to suture the corneoscleral section. The risk of having a large section such as expulsive hemorrhage, etc. are also reduced. This foldable glued IOL also has postoperative advantages of doing away with all complications associated with larger wounds such as postoperative wound leak, shallow AC, etc. as well as decreases the astigmatism associated with a large wound. To be able to perform this technique with ease, it is imperative that the surgeon becomes familiar with the handshake technique.

REFERENCES

1. Agarwal A, Kumar DA, Jacob S, Baid C, Agarwal A, Srinivasan S. Fibrin glue-assisted sutureless posterior chamber intraocular lens implantation in eyes with deficient posterior capsules. J Cataract Refract Surg. 2008;34(9):1433-8.
2. Kumar DA, Agarwal A, Prakash G, Jacob S, Saravanan Y, Agarwal A. Glued posterior chamber IOL in eyes with deficient capsular support: a retrospective analysis of 1-year postoperative outcomes. Eye (Lond). 2010;24(7):1143-8.
3. Prakash G, Kumar DA, Jacob S, Kumar KS, Agarwal A, Agarwal A. Anterior segment optical coherence tomography-aided diagnosis and primary posterior chamber intraocular lens implantation with fibrin glue in traumatic phacocele with scleral perforation. J Cataract Refract Surg. 2009;35(4):782-4.
4. Prakash G, Jacob S, Kumar DA, Narsimhan S, Agarwal A, Agarwal A. Femtosecond assisted keratoplasty with fibrin glue-assisted sutureless posterior chamber lens implantation: a new triple procedure. J Cataract Refract Surg. 2009;35(6):973-9.
5. Nair V, Kumar DA, Prakash G, Jacob S, Agarwal A, Agarwal A. Bilateral spontaneous in-the-bag anterior subluxation of PC IOL managed with glued IOL technique: A case report. Eye Contact Lens. 2009;35(4):215-7.
6. Agarwal A, Kumar DA, Prakash G, et al. Fibrin glue-assisted sutureless posterior chamber intraocular lens implantation in eyes with deficient posterior capsules [Reply to letter]. J Cataract Refract Surg. 2009;35(5):795-6.
7. Kumar DA, Agarwal A, Jacob S, Prakash G, Agarwal A, Sivagnanam S. Repositioning of the dislocated intraocular lens with sutureless 20-gauge vitrectomy Retina. 2010;30(4):682-7.
8. Kumar DA, Agarwal A, Prakash G, Jacob S. Managing total aniridia with aphakia using a glued iris prosthesis. J Cataract Refract Surg. 2010;36(5):864-5.
9. Kumar DA, Agarwal A, Gabor SG, et al. Sutureless sclera fixated posterior chamber intraocular lens. Letter to editor. J Cataract Refract Surg. 2011;37(11):2089-90.

CHAPTER 8

Modifications in the Glued Intraocular Lens Technique

Priya Narang, George Beiko, Toshihiko Ohta, Amar Agarwal

INTRODUCTION

Since its invention, the glued IOL technique[1-3] has continuously evolved and has now reached a stage where it is accepted worldwide. Various modifications have come up which have rectified and improvised each and every step of the surgery.

NO-ASSISTANT TECHNIQUE

'No-assistant technique'[4,5] is an effort to decrease the dependence on the assistant and make it more surgeon dependent. This technique is an attempt to make the process of 'externalization of haptics' which is considered to be the most technically demanding part of the surgery; more easy and feasible. The concept of no-assistant technique was conceptualized by one of us (PN).

Three Hands in Glued Intraocular Lens Surgery

Normally in a glued IOL surgery, the assistant holds the leading haptic while the surgeon engages in the externalization of the trailing haptic. A definite part of surgical expertise is required for the assistant to hold the haptic properly. Undue pressure on the haptic causes it to flatten which is then difficult to tuck. Inability of the assistant to hold the leading haptic along the correct plane causes IOL torsion while externalization and renders the procedure difficult at times.

Physics

The entire technique works on the simple principle of physics—the vector forces. The mid-pupillary plane is the major contributor to the success of this technique.

Normal Scenario (Fig. 8.1A)

After externalization of the leading haptic, there is a tendency of the haptic to slip back into the anterior chamber due to vector forces acting along the axis of the IOL. Green arrow indicates the vector forces.

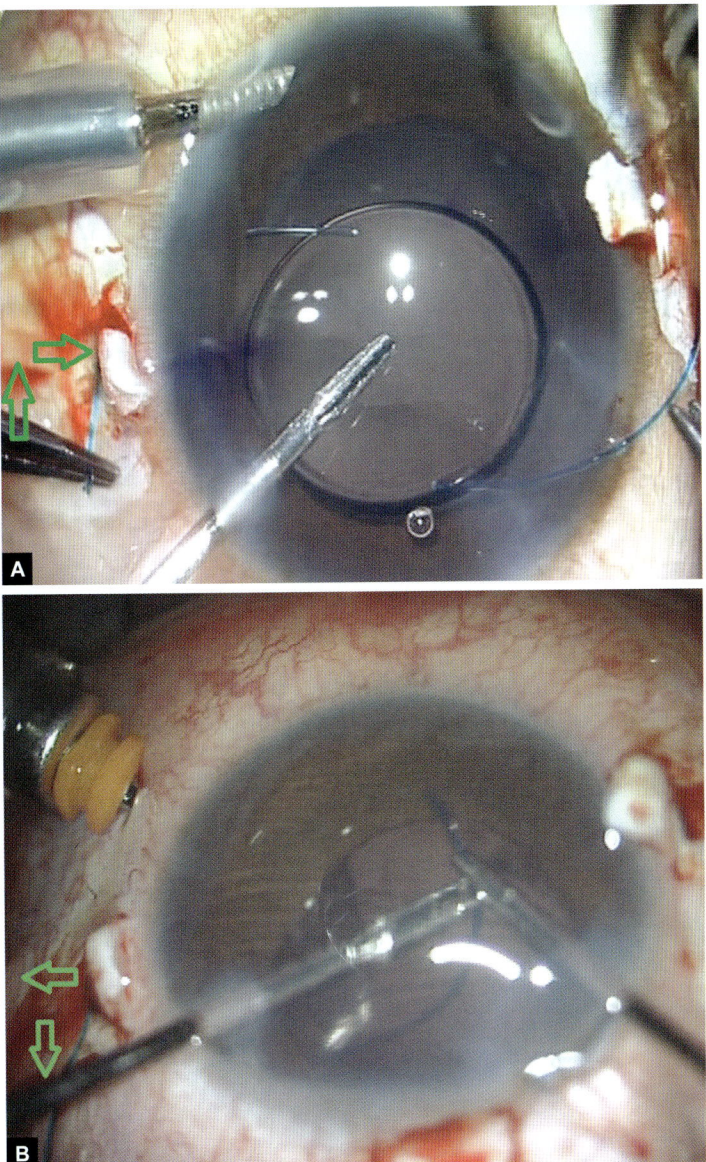

Figs 8.1A and B Physics in no-assistant technique. Green arrows indicate the vector forces. (A) Normal glued IOL surgery-At this stage, the assistant surgeon needs to hold the haptic because it tends to slip back into the eye as the vector forces are acting along the axis of the IOL (inwards); (B) No-assistant technique—as the IOL crosses the mid pupillary plane, the vector forces act in a way (outwards) which ensures that the haptic does not slip back into anterior chamber

No-assistant Technique (Fig. 8.1B)

When the trailing haptic crosses the mid-pupillary plane and is nearly at 6 O'clock position, the vector forces act in a way that causes further extrusion of the leading haptic from the sclerotomy site with virtually no chance of slippage of leading haptic into the anterior chamber.

SURGICAL TECHNIQUE

As usual, two partial scleral thickness flaps 2.5 by 2.5 mm are made 180° opposite followed by introduction of infusion in to the eye by either an AC maintainer or a Trocar cannula. A sclerotomy wound is created with a 20 G needle approximately 1.0 mm from the limbus beneath the scleral flaps. Vitrectomy is then done from the same sclerotomy site with a 23 G cutter.

Corneal tunnel is fashioned followed by a side port entry. The IOL is loaded and the tip of the haptic is slightly brought out from the cartridge. The loaded cartridge is then entered into the eye while the glued IOL forceps is introduced from the sclerotomy site. The tip of the haptic is then grasped and the IOL is slowly unfolded (Figs 8.2A to D). When the entire IOL has unfolded, the leading haptic is pulled and externalized.

The trailing haptic is then grasped with the glued IOL forceps while the left hand still holds onto the leading haptic. The trailing haptic is then moved inferiorly up to 6 O'clock position. This ensures that no external forces are acting on the leading haptic which causes it to slip inside. The surgeon leaves the leading haptic and then introduces the glued IOL forceps from the side port incision. The tip of the trailing haptic is then transferred to the second forceps (Figs 8.3A to C). Now the surgeon enters the eye from the other sclerotomy site with the Glued IOL forceps and catches the tip of the trailing haptic using the handshake technique. The trailing haptic is then pulled out and externalized (Fig. 8.3D). The haptics are then tucked in the scleral pockets and vitrectomy is done at the sclerotomy site. The infusion is stopped and the glue is applied beneath the scleral flaps and the corneal incision sites are also sealed with glue.

Advantages

- Fast and easy
- Totally surgeon dependent. Manipulation and externalization of haptics becomes technically very handy.

Summary

'No-assistant technique' is an armamentarium in the hands of the glued IOL surgeon as it enables the surgeon to externalize the haptics without the need of any assistant to hold on to the leading haptic. It renders the surgery more 'surgeon' dependent rather than 'assistant' dependent.

Modifications in the Glued Intraocular Lens Technique

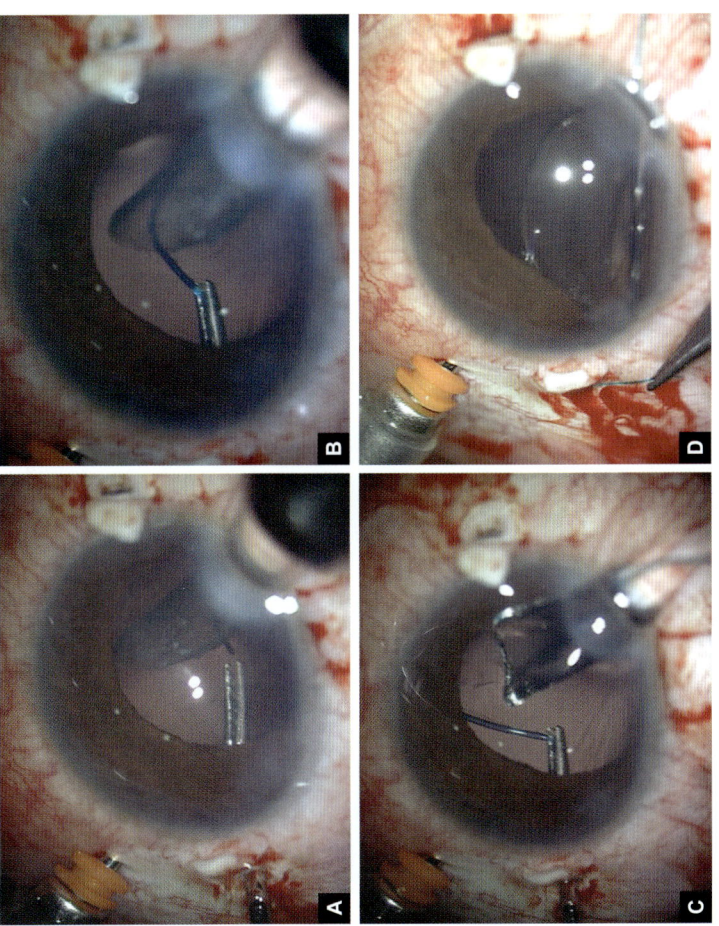

Figs 8.2A to D Leading haptic externalization in no-assistant technique. (A) Tip of the leading haptic about to be grasped with glued IOL forceps; (B) Tip of the leading haptic caught with glued IOL forceps; (C) Haptic still caught with the forceps while IOL is being injected. Note the haptic is not externalized; (D) Leading haptic externalized after the entire IOL has unfolded. The trailing haptic is still outside the corneal incision. Once externalized the surgeon holds the haptic so that it does not slip back

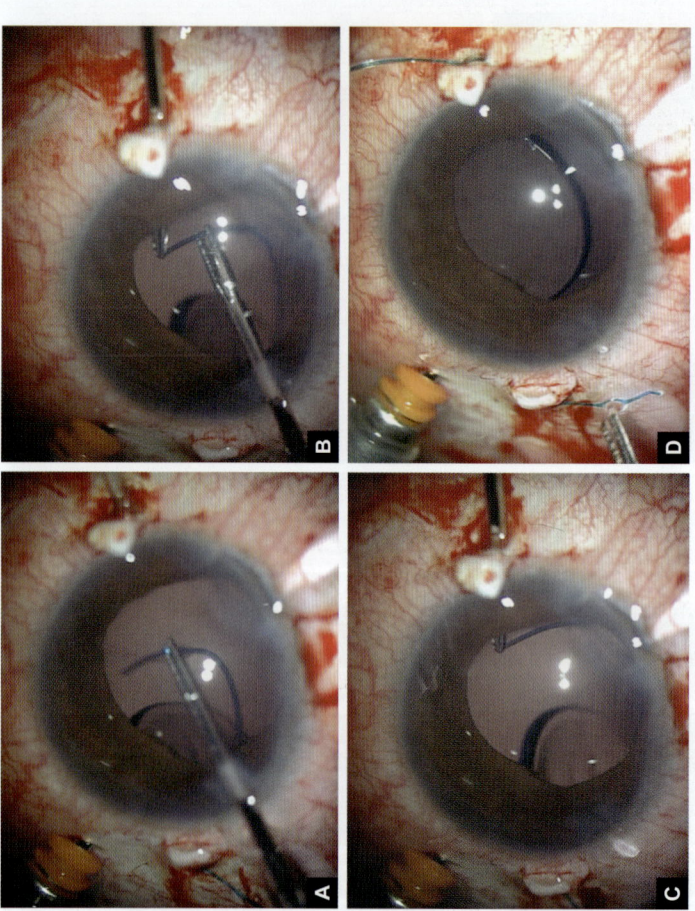

Figs 8.3A to D Trailing haptic externalization in no-assistant technique. (A) The trailing haptic is moved inferiorly up to 6 O'clock position. This way the physics of vector forces come into play and the leading haptic now does not slip back into the eye. Surgeon leaves the leading haptic, and a glued IOL forceps introduced from the side port incision grasps the trailing haptic; (B) The tip of trailing haptic is transferred to the second forceps using the handshake technique; (C) Tip of the trailing haptic is caught with the glued IOL forceps; (D) Trailing haptic is externalized. Finally, both haptics are externalized without the help of an assistant

Vertical Glued Intraocular Lens

One should measure the horizontal white to white diameter of the cornea. If it is more than 11 mm one can do a vertical glued IOL as the vertical diameter will always be shorter and one will have more haptic to tuck. Vertical glued IOL was started by *Jeevan Ladi* from India, and the scleral flaps are made at 12 and 6 O'clock position with the surgeon sitting temporally.

Needle-Guided Intrascleral Fixation of Posterior Chamber Intraocular Lens for Aphakia Correction

Iñaki Rodríguez-Agirretxe and others from Instituto Clínico Quirúrgico de Oftalmología, Vizcaya, Spain came out with this concept. A 3-piece IOL is inserted into the anterior chamber and the IOL is then rotated so the tip of the haptic to be externalized faces the scleral flap. Using a 25-gauge needle, a straight sclerotomy is made 1.0 mm from the sclerocorneal limbus. The haptic is guided into the needle and the needle withdrawn. This ensures that the haptic is also withdrawn with the needle. Then intrascleral haptic fixation can be done.

BEIKO AND STEINERT'S MODIFICATION

Roger Steinert and George Beiko suggested the use of silicon tires or plugs to prevent slippage of leading haptic in to the eye.[6] The technique of glued IOL requires an assistant to hold the haptics of the IOL once they have been externalized through the sclerotomies. If an assistant is not available, it is likely that the externalized haptic will be pulled into the eye once the second haptic is externalized. In order to prevent the migration of the first haptic into the eye, it is possible to use a silicone tire or a plug (Figs 8.4A to D). The silicone tires are readily available from a Mackool capsular support system (Impex surgical) or MST capsular support (Microsurgical technology Inc.). Placing the silicone tire on the haptic provides support for the haptic while the entire procedure is performed.

Choice of Tissue Glue

George Beiko has used both TISSEEL (Baxter Corp.) and Evicel (Ethicon Inc.). The two tissue glues are similar; TISSEEL contains aprotinin, an antifibrinolytic agent, while EVICEL is manufactured without plasminogen and as such does not contain an antifibrinogen agent. There is a difference in the preparation of the agents. EVICEL is stored frozen; once thawed, it has to be used within 24 hours if kept at room temperature or within 30 days if stored in a refrigerator. TISSEEL is also stored frozen; it has to be thawed, and then warmed to 33 to 37°C and has to be used within 4 hours of preparation.

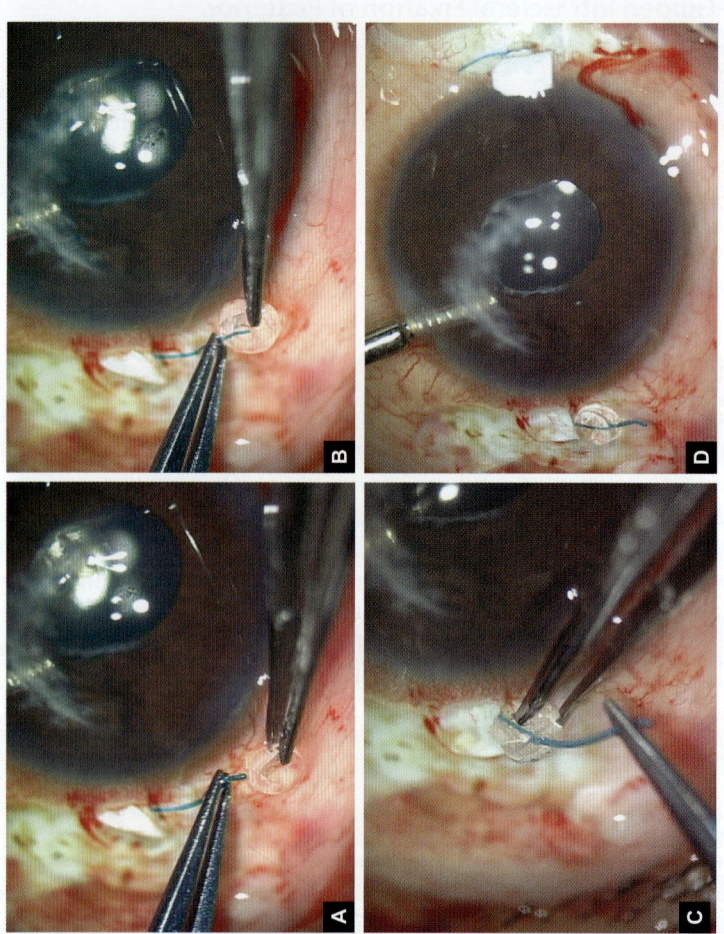

Figs 8.4A to D Beiko's modification. (A and B) Haptic passed through the narrow opening in the silicone tire of an iris hook; (C) Haptic passed fully; (D) Silicone tire of iris hook prevents the haptic from slipping back into the vitreous cavity

Choice of Forceps Tips

23 G instruments are recommended by Beiko. The tips can be either ridged or smooth. The problem with ridged tips is that they can result in crinkling of the haptics. Crinkling of haptics, especially prolene haptics, results in weakening and the haptics can easily break. Broken haptics can be a problem as the amount available for threading into the scleral tunnel will be limited.

TOSHIHIKO OHTA'S Y-FIXATION TECHNIQUE

Toshihiko Ohta from Japan started a simplified and safer method of sutureless intrascleral posterior chamber intraocular lens fixation. This is called the Y-fixation technique (Figs 8.5A to G).

Technique

Under peribulbar anesthesia, a 5 mm conjunctival peritomy is done at the 2 O'clock and 8 O'clock positions (Figs 8.6A to I). A reference marker and Y marker (Duckworth and Kent, England) are used for marking (Figs 8.7 and 8.8). Then two Y-shaped incisions are made 2 mm from the limbus exactly 180 degrees apart diagonally. An infusion cannula or anterior chamber maintainer is inserted. To prevent interference with the creation of the Y-shaped incision, the infusion cannula should be positioned at 5 O'clock. Anterior vitrectomy is performed, if necessary. A 23-gauge MVR knife is used to perform a sclerotomy parallel to the iris at the Y-shaped incision, and a scleral tunnel is made parallel to the limbus at the end of the Y-shaped incision. Next, a 2.4 to 3.0 mm keratome is used to make a corneal incision at 10 O'clock for injector-assisted IOL implantation. A standard 3-piece IOL is implanted with an injector and the trailing haptic is left outside the corneal incision. The leading haptic is then grasped at its tip with a 25-gauge IOL haptic gripping forceps (Eye technology, England), pulled through the sclerotomy, and externalized on the left side. After the trailing haptic is inserted into the anterior chamber with a forceps, a U-shaped hook (Duckworth and Kent, England) is used to guide it to the center of the pupil (U-shaped hook technique) (Figs 8.9 and 8.10). Then the tip of the haptic is grasped with the 25-gauge forceps, pulled through the second sclerotomy, and externalized on the right side. The tip of the IOL haptic is subsequently inserted into the limbus-parallel scleral tunnel with a forceps, after which the IOL is positioned and centered. A single 8-0 nylon suture is used to fix the haptic to the scleral bed in order to prevent it shifting immediately after surgery and the incision is closed with 8-0 Vicryl. After the incision is closed completely and the haptic embedded into the sclera, the anterior chamber maintainer or infusion cannula is removed. Finally, the conjunctiva is closed with 8-0 Vicryl.

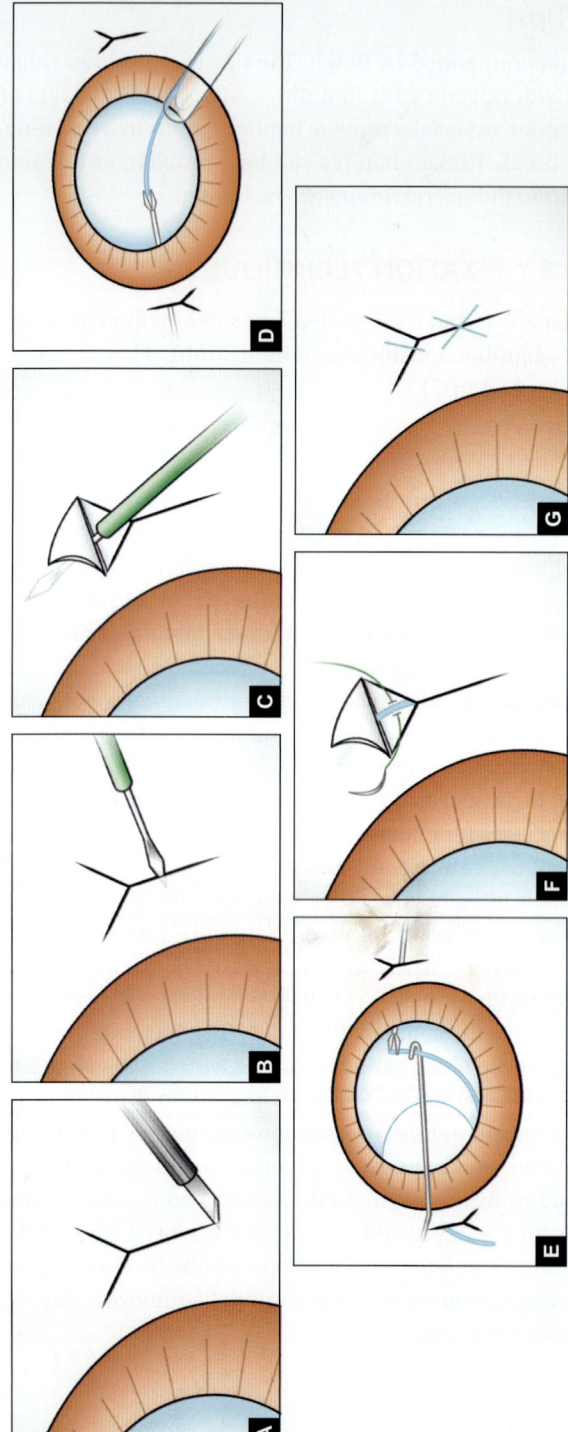

Figs 8.5A to G Illustrations depicting Ohta's Y-fixation technique. (A) A Y-shaped incision is made 2 mm from the limbus; (B) A 23-gauge MVR knife performs sclerotomy parallel to the iris; (C) The 23-gauge MVR knife creates a scleral tunnel; (D) Leading haptic caught with the 25-gauge forceps; (E) A U-shaped hook is used to guide the IOL haptic to the center of the pupil. Then the tip of the IOL haptic is grasped with a 25-gauge forceps and pulled through the second sclerotomy; (F) An 8-0 nylon suture is placed in the scleral bed to prevent shifting of IOL immediately after surgery; (G) The sclera is sutured with 8-0 Vicryl, the incision is completely closed, and the haptic is embedded into the sclera

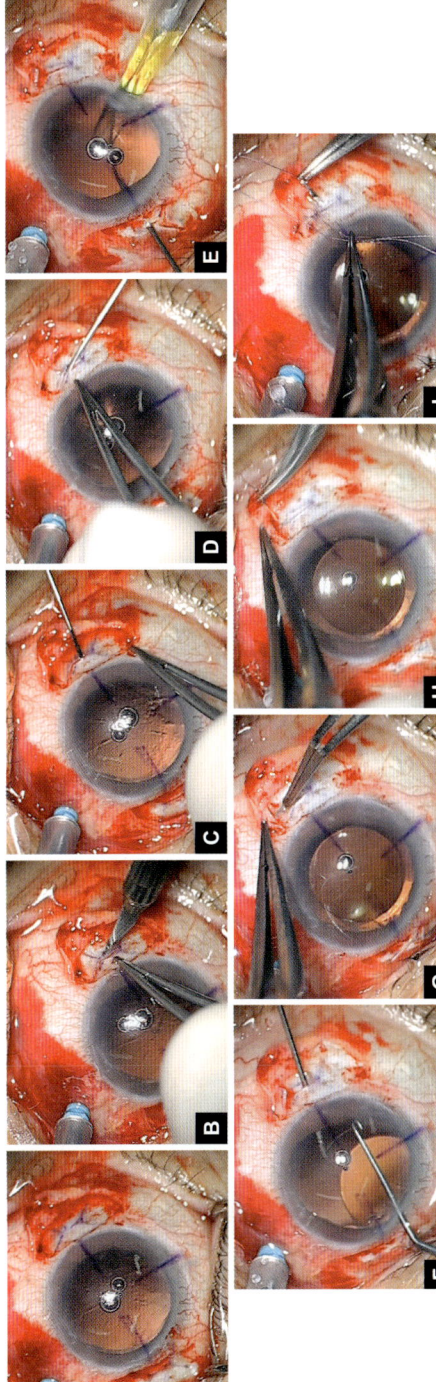

Figs 8.6A to I Surgical technique of Ohta's Y-fixation technique. (A) A 5 mm conjunctival peritomy is done at 2 O'clock and 8 O'clock positions, a reference marker and Y-marker are used for marking; (B) A Y-shaped incision is made 2 mm from the limbus; (C) A 23-gauge MVR knife is used to perform a sclerotomy parallel to the iris; (D) The 23-gauge MVR knife creates a scleral tunnel parallel to the limbus at the end of the Y-shaped incision; (E) The leading haptic is grasped at the tip with a 25-gauge forceps and pulled through the sclerotomy; (F) A U-shaped hook is used to guide the IOL haptic to the center of the pupil. Then the tip of the IOL haptic is grasped with a 25-gauge forceps and pulled through the second sclerotomy; (G) The tip of the IOL haptic is inserted into the limbus-parallel scleral tunnel with a forceps; (H) An 8-0 nylon suture is placed in the scleral bed to prevent the IOL shifting immediately after surgery; (I) The sclera is sutured with 8-0 Vicryl, the incision is completely closed, and the haptic is embedded into the sclera

Management of PHACO Complications: Newer Techniques

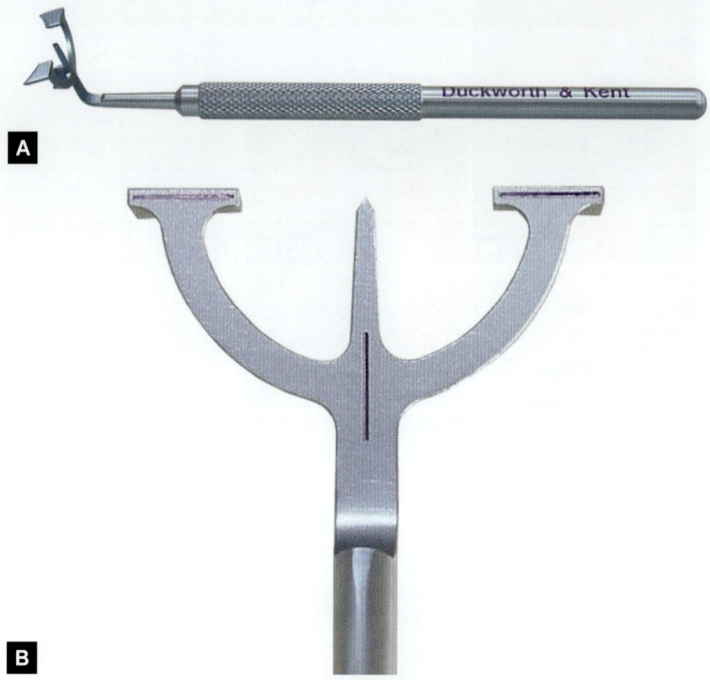

Figs 8.7A and B Ohta's reference marker for the intrascleral IOL fixation technique. (Duckworth & Kent, England)

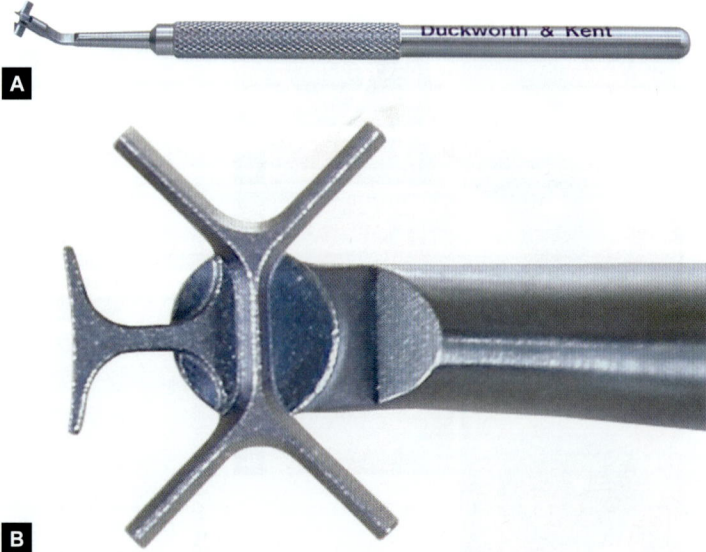

Figs 8.8A and B Ohta's Y-marker for the intrascleral IOL fixation technique. (Duckworth & Kent, England)

Modifications in the Glued Intraocular Lens Technique

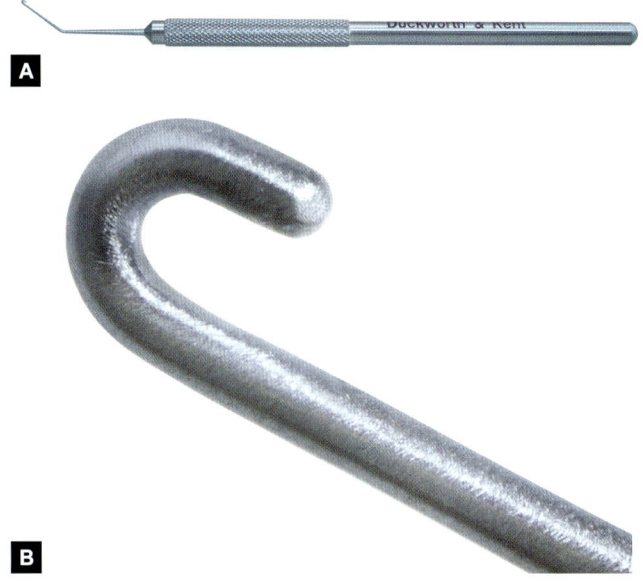

Figs 8.9A and B U-shaped hook for the intrascleral IOL fixation technique. (Duckworth & Kent, England)

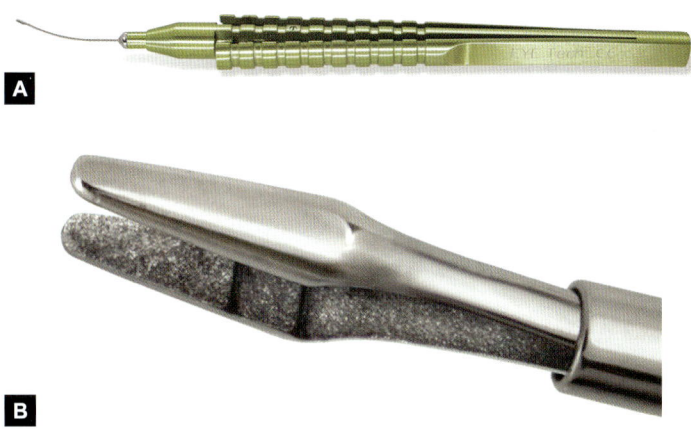

Figs 8.10A and B Ohta's IOL haptic gripping forceps (25 G). (Eye technology, England)

Results

This technique was used in 44 eyes of 42 patients. No intraoperative complications occurred. All IOLs were stable and centered at the end of surgery. Although IOL decentration was subsequently observed in 2 eyes due to ocular contusion, correction was done without difficulty. There was no decline of best-corrected visual acuity (BCVA) except in one eye with postoperative retinal detachment. In 5 eyes with a dislocated IOL, the same IOL was used again. As for postoperative complications, compared with suture fixation, there was significantly less IOL decentration and tilt. Astigmatism of the IOL was also significantly less marked than with suture fixation, showing virtually no difference from intracapsular fixation.

DISCUSSION

Gabor, et al. described a technique for intrascleral fixation of both haptics in the ciliary sulcus by means of a parallel scleral tunnel, with a 24-gauge needle being used to create a straight sclerotomy. However, extracting the haptic is difficult, it can only be done with a 3-piece IOL, and closure is problematic. Agarwal, et al. used a 22-gauge needle to create a straight sclerotomy and bioadhesive to attach the haptics and to glue the scleral flaps and overlying conjunctiva. However, their technique has problems with regard to closure and postoperative hypotony, using fibrin glue, and the creation of a lamellar scleral flap. The Y-Fixation technique is a new intrascleral IOL fixation method that does not involve complicated manipulation and achieves safer sutureless fixation. With the Y-Fixation technique, a Y-shaped incision is made in the sclera and a 23-gauge MVR knife is used to create the sclerotomy instead of a needle. The Y-shaped incision eliminates the need to raise a lamellar scleral flap, while performing sclerotomy with the 23-gauge MVR knife simplifies extraction of the haptic and greatly improves wound closure.

SUMMARY

The Y-fixation technique is simpler and safer than the other intrascleral IOL fixation techniques. This technique is a new generation secondary IOL implantation method that achieves both anatomical and optical stability. Further development of this technique can be expected in the future.

PROBLEMS WITH THE GLUED INTRAOCULAR LENS TECHNIQUE AND THEIR SOLUTIONS

1. **Hypotony:** Hypotony, sometimes severe (IOP 2–4 mm Hg) can be a common denominator in some cases. We need to learn how to solve this problem of hypotony.
    - Fill the AC with air. Don't over fill it too much as that pushes the iris way down. Just have enough air in the AC. Now inject some balanced salt solution (BSS) inside the eye if you feel the eye is hypotonic. The hypotony occurs not due to the sclerotomies or 26-gauge tunnels. This can happen if you are not using glue but with glue hypotony will not occur due to these factors.

- At the end of the case once you have stuck the flaps and conjunctiva with glue, injected the subconjunctival injection and removed the speculum, check if the eye is hypotonic. If you feel the eye is soft, inject immediately some BSS through the clear corneal incision till the eye becomes solid. What happens now is that air is in the AC and the fluid you inject will go through the pupil into the vitreous cavity and distend the eye.
- Hypotony is due to the fact that we have removed vitreous and sometimes the fluid is not there. Point B will solve it.
- Postoperatively, if you see hypotony, put the patient on systemic steroids and it will resolve. But with point B followed of BSS injected at the end of the case into the AC, hypotony will generally be not observed.
- Do not leave an eye hypotonic at the end of the surgery which is the key to successful surgery.

2. **3-piece IOL deformation:** Any 3-piece IOL can be used. One main issue of deformation is if the tip of the haptic is not caught. If the haptic is slightly deformed you can straighten it outside the eye using two tying forceps once the haptic is externalized. If you have externalized the haptics and got quite a bit of haptic out and if the tip is deformed and tucking is difficult then just take a scissor and cut the tip. It is like a thread being passed through a needle. Sometimes the thread tip gets deformed and does not pass through the eye of the needle. In such a case, you just break the tip of the thread and then it passes through easily.

3. **Too much haptic externalized; haptics too long to tuck into the tunnels:** This is very easy to treat. Just chop the haptics if they are too long after externalization. Let's say you have 5 mm haptic externalized and it is too long, then just take a scissor and cut the extra portion and tuck the remaining haptic. Same will happen when you operate a micro cornea eye with a coloboma. They may require a glued IOL.

4. **Concerns of late redislocation:** If the surgery is done well you will not get a dislocation even after several years. Early dislocations within a month highlights the fact that the haptics were not tucked well or the amount of haptic tucked was not enough, etc. If the haptics are tucked and glued well there is no way that haptic can come out. The issue is not the same with sutures as it can break.

CONCLUSION

Various modifications have been proposed for the intrascleral haptic fixation of a PCIOL and glued IOL techniques. Each technique has its own pros and cons. It is up to the surgeon to choose which technique is the best.

REFERENCES

1. Agarwal A, Kumar DA, Jacob S, Baid C, Agarwal A, Srinivasan S. Fibrin glue-assisted sutureless posterior chamber intraocular lens implantation in eyes with deficient posterior capsules. J Cataract Refract Surg. 2008;34(9):1433-8.
2. Kumar DA, Agarwal A, Prakash G, Jacob S, Saravanan Y, Agarwal A. Glued posterior chamber IOL in eyes with deficient capsular support: a retrospective analysis of 1-year post-operative outcomes. Eye (Lond). 2010;24(7):1143-8.
3. Narang P, Narang S. Glue-assisted intrascleral fixation of posterior chamber intraocular lens. Indian J Ophthal. 2013;61(4):163-7. doi: 10.4103/0301-4738.112160.
4. Narang P. Modified method of haptic externalization of posterior chamber intraocular lens in fibrin glue-assisted intrascleral fixation: No-assistant technique. J Cataract Refract Surg. 2013;39:4-7.
5. Narang P. Postoperative analysis of glued intrascleral fixation of intraocular lens and comparison of intraoperative parameters and visual outcome with 2 methods of haptic externalization. J Cataract Refract Surg. 2013;39:1118-9.
6. Beiko G, Steinert R. Modification of externalized haptic support of glued intraocular lens technique. J Cataract Refract Surg. 2013;39:323-9.

CHAPTER 9

Intraocular Lens Scaffold

Priya Narang, Amar Agarwal

INTRODUCTION

A breach in the continuity of the posterior capsule is a cause of concern. Posterior capsular rupture (PCR) is a dreaded complication of cataract surgery; it jeopardises the chances of inserting a posterior chamber lens and therefore obtaining the ideal optical correction. The purpose of modern cataract surgery is to maintain the integrity of the posterior capsule, not only to support the intraocular lens (IOL), but to diminish the incidence of retinal complications like cystoid macular edema and retinal detachment.

Posterior capsular rupture (PCR) develops most frequently during removal of the last nuclear fragment following a transient postocclusion surge, especially when dealing with a dense nucleus.[1] Early recognition and proper management of PCR are important as they limit the size of the capsule tear, minimize vitreous loss, and avert the disaster of a dropped nucleus. The conventional management consists of prevention of mixture of cortical matter with vitreous, dry aspiration, and anterior vitrectomy. In addition, during phacoemulsification low flow rate, high vacuum, and low ultrasound are advocated if a posterior capsule tear occurs.

The IOL scaffold procedure[2,3] is intended for use in cases where PCR occurs with a nonemulsified, moderate to soft nucleus. A three piece foldable IOL acts as a scaffold or a barrier to compartmentalize the anterior and posterior chambers, thereby preventing the vitreous prolapse, vitreous hydration and nucleus drop.

SURGICAL TECHNIQUE

The surgery is performed under peribulbar anesthesia. Upon recognition of a PCR, dispersive viscoelastic is injected to seal the capsular break from the side port incision without withdrawal of the phaco probe. After adequate sealing of the rent, the phaco probe is withdrawn and dispersive OVD is used to levitate and bring all the nuclear remnants into the anterior chamber (Fig. 9.1A). In cases of small PCR's, the tear is converted into a posterior capsulorhexis; whereas in cases of large tears it is difficult to do so. A 23/25 G vitrectomy probe is introduced with

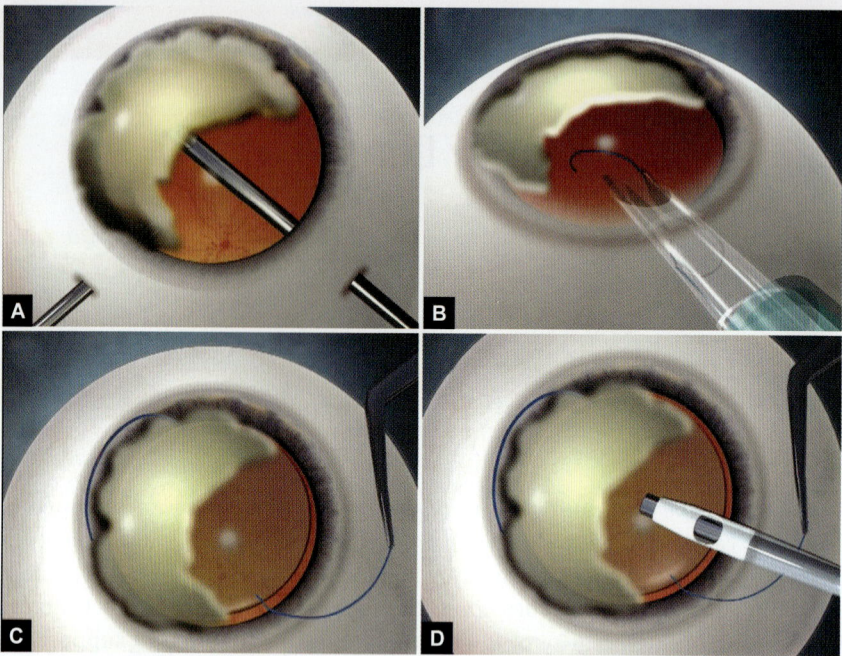

Figs 9.1A to D Animated demonstration of IOL scaffold. (A) Nuclear remnants are lifted into the anterior chamber; (B) A 3-piece foldable intraocular lens (IOL) is being injected beneath the nuclear remnant; (C) Trailing haptic left extruded from the corneal incision; (D) Phacoemulsification probe is being introduced above the IOL

high cutting rate and adequate suction parameters. The infusion needle can be used to maintain the anterior chamber during vitrectomy; care being taken so that the fluid does not push the nuclear fragments down. The direction of the flow should be beneath the nuclear fragment towards the pupillary area. The pupillary area is cleared of vitreous and the presence of any strand is confirmed with the use of triamcinolone acetonide 0.5 cc injection. A 3-piece foldable IOL is injected beneath the nuclear fragment in a way that the leading haptic is guided and placed above the capsulorhexis while the trailing haptic is left extruded at the corneal incision (Figs 9.1B and C; Figs 9.3A and B). The phacoemulsification probe is introduced into the eye and the nuclear fragments are emulsified (Fig. 9.1D, Fig. 9.2A; Figs 9.3C and D). Using a dialler in the nondominant hand, the surgeon maneuvers the optic-haptic junction on the trailing haptic side so that the IOL blocks the pupil (Fig. 9.2 B). Keeping the trailing haptic outside the incision enables adjustment of the IOL position in case if the nucleus rotates thus reducing the risk of IOL drop. Any residual cortex is then removed using the vitrectomy probe in suction mode with low aspiration. The IOL is maneuvered over the capsular remnants in the ciliary sulcus (Fig. 9.2C and D; Figs 9.3E and F). If the capsular support is inadequate, a glued IOL procedure is performed. The

Intraocular Lens Scaffold

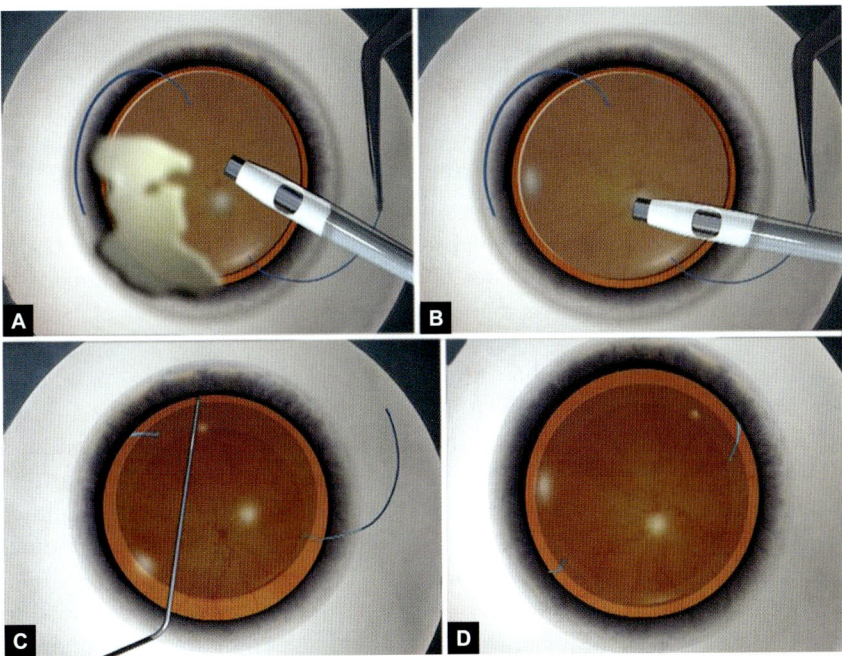

Figs 9.2A to D Animated demonstration of IOL scaffold. (A) Nuclear remnants are being emulsified; (B) Phacoemulsification complete; (C) Intraocular lens (IOL) is being dialed into sulcus; (D) Well placed IOL above capsulorhexis

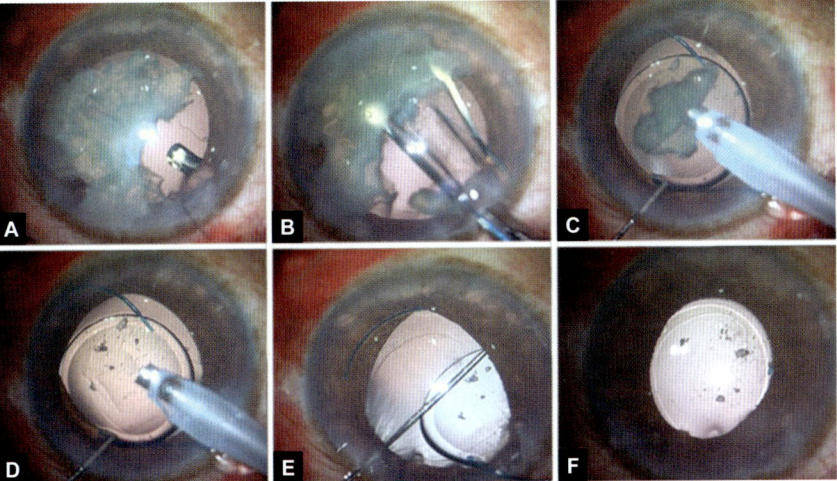

Figs 9.3A to F Clinical pictures of IOL scaffold technique. (A) Vitrectomy is being done beneath the nuclear fragments; (B) A 3-piece foldable injected beneath the nuclear remnants; (C) Phacoemulsification is being done. The IOL acts as a scaffold and prevents the drop of nuclear material in the vitreous cavity; (D) Phacoemulsification complete; (E) Intraocular lens (IOL) is being dialed into sulcus; (F) Intraocular lens (IOL) in sulcus.

infusion cannula/anterior chamber maintainer is removed, and the trailing haptic is then dialled into position above the capsulorhexis and the stability of the IOL checked. The incisions are hydrated and checked for stability.

DISCUSSION

Posterior capsular rupture is a known complication of cataract surgery. The incidence of this complication is higher amongst trainees but it can occur in the hands of experienced surgeon's too.[4,5] Loss of vitreous causes significant ocular morbidity and its appropriate management is an important aspect of cataract surgery.[6]

After the posterior capsule rupture, removal of residual lens material is a challenging but important goal. Sequential, interdependent strategies to accomplish this include the Viscoat PAL, the Viscoat Trap, bimanual pars plana anterior vitrectomy, and bimanual irrigation-aspiration of cortex. Once brought into the anterior chamber, the nucleus can be removed either with phacoemulsification above a Sheet's glide, or by converting to a manual extracapsular cataract extraction approach.[A]

The dispersive viscoelastic serves as an effective barrier to vitreous prolapse while preventing posterior dislocation of lens material. Viscodissection or manually moving the remaining lens material up out of the remaining capsule and into the anterior chamber can be done from where it can be safely emulsified and aspirated.[A,B] A pars plana sclerotomy to inject the supplemental supporting viscoelastic behind the nucleus, and then using the cannula tip to elevate the nuclear fragments forward through the pupil, under direct microscopic visualization.[A]

Intraocular lens scaffold is a technique aimed at preventing complications and achieving a successful visual outcome after posterior capsular rupture. As the IOL is inserted through the existing corneal incision, this technique has an advantage of maintaining anterior chamber stability and the intraocular pressure (IOP) while preserving the astigmatic benefits of sutureless, small incision surgery.

As the name suggests, a 3-piece IOL acts as a temporary platform or a scaffold, preventing nuclear fragments from falling into the vitreous cavity.

The technique can be used after the nuclear fragments are brought into the anterior chamber, but it should be limited to the management of PCR in eyes with soft to moderate nuclei, considering the risk of corneal damage in cases of hard cataract.

The advantages with this technique are that it establishes a physical barrier to nucleus drop without any need to enlarge the phacoemulsification incision. Also there is no need for sutures that might induce postoperative astigmatism. Preventing nucleus fragments from falling into the vitreous eliminates added risks from secondary surgery for large dropped fragment removal.

CONCLUSION

In conclusion, IOL scaffold can be done successfully with low complication rates with the aid of three piece IOL serving as a scaffold for the nuclear remnants in patients with posterior capsular rupture.

REFERENCES

1. Soon-Phaik Chee. Pseudo anterior capsule barrier for the management of posterior capsule rupture. J Cataract Refract Surg. 2012;38:1309-15.
2. Kumar DA, Agarwal A, Prakash G, et al. IOL scaffold technique for posterior capsular rupture. J Refract Surg. 2012;28:314-5.
3. Narang P, Agarwal A, Kumar DA, et al. Clinical outcomes of intraocular scaffold lens surgery. A one year study. Ophthalmology. 2013;120:2442-8.
4. Haripriya A, Chang D, Mascarenhas R, Shekhar M. Complication rates of phacoemulsification and manual small-incision cataract surgery at Aravind Eye Hospital. J Cataract Refract Surg. 2012;38:1360-9.
5. Unal M, Yucel I, Sarıcı A, Artunay O, Devranoglu K, Akar Y, Altın M. Phacoemulsification with topical anesthesia: resident experience. J Cataract Refract Surg. 2006;32:1361-5.
6. Reddy MK. Complications of cataract surgery. Indian J Ophthalmol. 1995;43:201-9.

SUGGESTED READING

A. Posterior Capsular Rupture During Cataract Surgery. Laura J Ronge Eye Net Magazine 200509.
B. B Michela Cimberle. Four strategies help manage posterior capsule rupture with nucleus present Viscoat PAL, the Viscoat "trap," bimanual pars plana vitrectomy and bimanual I & A can prevent dropped lens material. OSN Europe Asia Edition, October 2002.

CHAPTER 10

Glued Intraocular Lens Scaffold

Priya Narang, Amar Agarwal

INTRODUCTION

The first glued posterior chamber intraocular lens (IOL) implantation in an eye with a deficient capsule was done on 14th December 2007. Since 2007, a large number of cases have been done with this technique.[1-6] In 2011, we started a technique to prevent nuclear fragments from falling into the vitreous cavity called the IOL scaffold technique.[7] We hereby describe a technique that combines glued IOL with IOL scaffold thus creating an artificial posterior capsule in cases of posterior capsular rupture (PCR).

CONCEPT AND INDICATIONS

In the IOL scaffold technique, we implant a 3-piece foldable IOL above the iris or over the anterior capsule in cases of PCR. This prevents the nuclear pieces from descending into the vitreous, as the IOL acts as a scaffold or as a temporary platform. Once the nucleus is emulsified the same IOL can then be placed into the sulcus or glued to the sclera depending on the availability of the anterior capsule.

The problem is enhanced in cases of insufficient iris and anterior capsular support to facilitate the IOL scaffold technique. In such cases we cannot implant the IOL to support the nuclear pieces as then the IOL may sink. This can happen in cases like an iris coloboma (Fig. 10.1) in which a PCR has occurred and there is no capsular support at all. Alternatively in cases like a floppy iris where the iris is not taut enough to support the IOL or cases in which the pupil is very dilated and not constricting due to trauma and once again there is no capsular support.

SURGICAL TECHNIQUE

In cases of intraoperative PCR, the phacoemulsification procedure is withheld. The remaining nuclear pieces are brought into the anterior chamber. An infusion cannula is fixed and scleral flaps are fashioned as in glued IOL surgery (Fig. 10.2).

Glued Intraocular Lens Scaffold

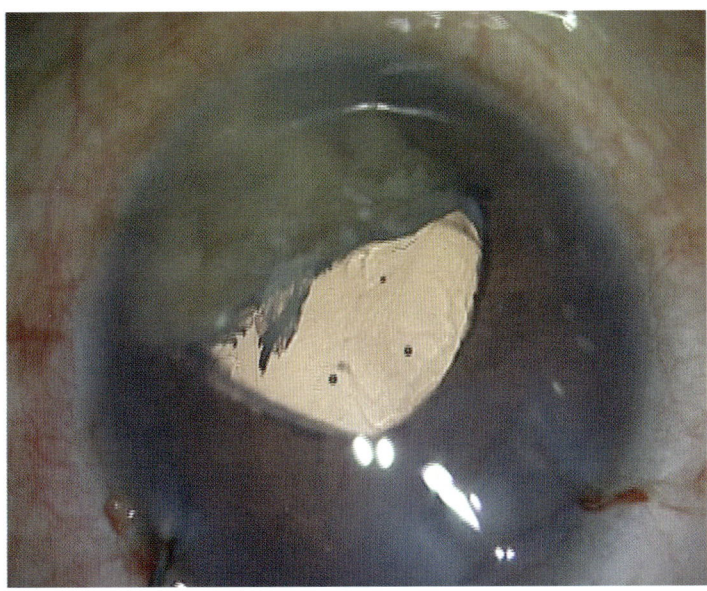

Fig. 10.1 Intraoperative posterior capsular rupture (PCR) noted. Nuclear pieces brought to the anterior chamber

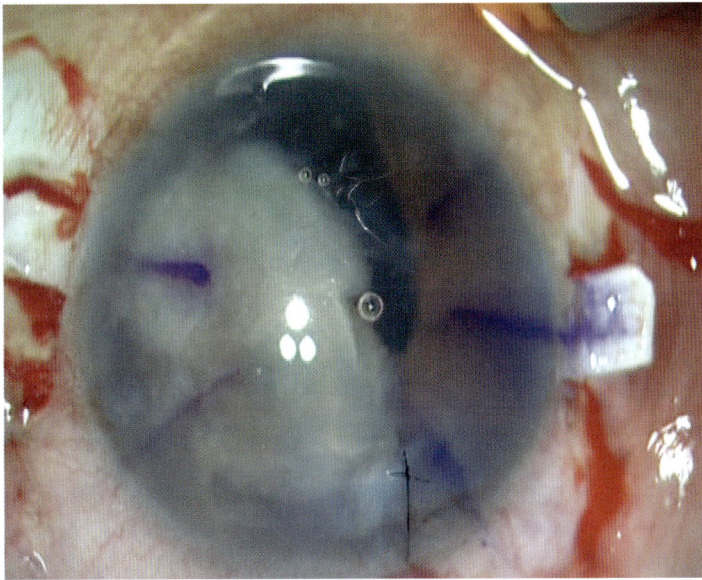

Fig. 10.2 Preparation for glued IOL surgery. Scleral flaps created. Note the infusion cannula through a trocar cannula

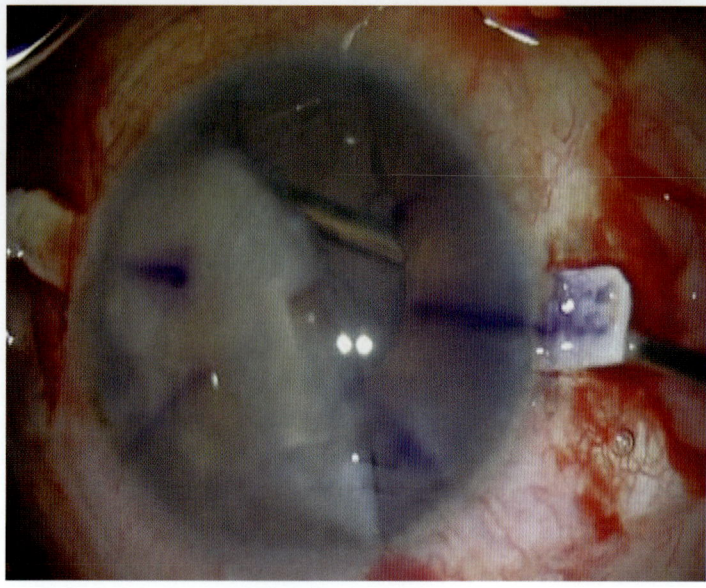

Fig. 10.3 Vitrectomy

Sclerotomy is then created with a 20 gauge needle approximately 1 mm behind the limbus under the scleral flaps. A 23 G vitrectomy probe is passed through the sclerotomy to perform vitrectomy so that all the tractional forces in the vitreous are nullified (Fig. 10.3). Vitrectomy is an essential step in the surgery as one can otherwise land up with a retinal detachment postoperatively.

The 3-piece foldable IOL is loaded onto the injector and the cartridge passed into the anterior chamber (AC) (Fig. 10.4). The haptic tip should be slightly out of the cartridge so that when one goes to grasp the haptic with the glued IOL forceps it is easy. The haptic tip is grasped with the glued IOL forceps and while the IOL is unfolded the haptic tip is still caught. The chances of the IOL falling down are not there as the haptic is caught with the forceps and the trailing haptic is still outside the clear corneal incision. Using the handshake technique, the trailing haptic is externalized (Fig. 10.5). If the nuclear pieces are occupying a lot of space in the AC, this maneuver is sometimes difficult. One should use viscoelastic to dislodge the pieces to the side to gain visualization.

A 26 G needle is used to create the Scharioth pocket and the haptics are tucked into the intrascleral pocket (Fig. 10.6). Phacoemulsification of the nuclear pieces is then performed (Fig. 10.7) as an artificial posterior capsule has been created using the combination of the glued IOL and the IOL scaffold technique (Fig. 10.8). This prevents the nuclear fragments from falling into the vitreous cavity. Finally air is injected into the AC and fibrin glue is used to seal the scleral flaps (Fig. 10.9).

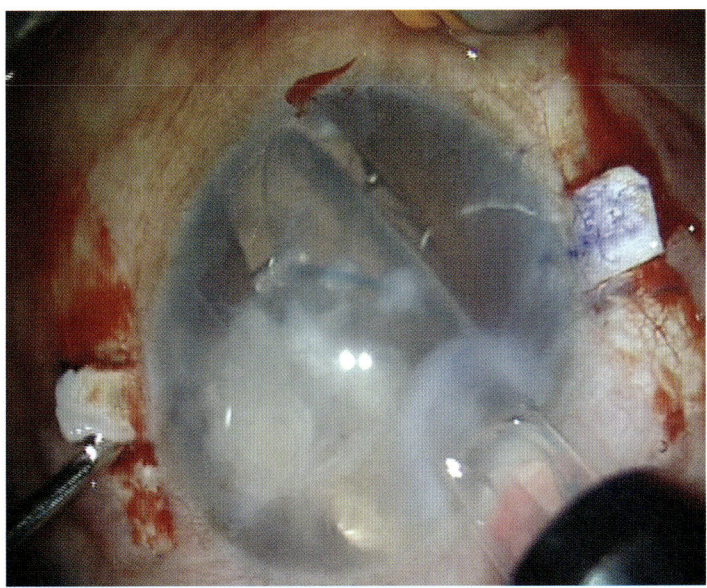

Fig. 10.4 3-piece foldable IOL implantation. Note the cartridge in the AC. Also note the haptic is slightly out of the cartridge so that it is easy for the glued IOL forceps to grasp the tip of the haptic

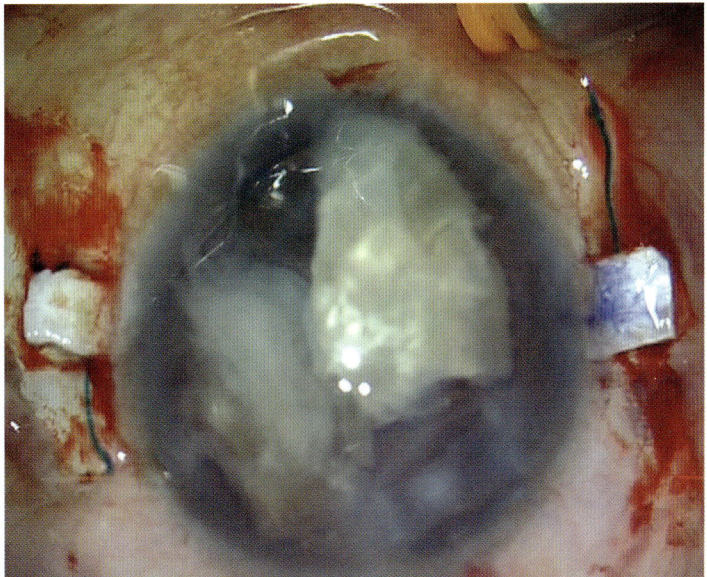

Fig. 10.5 Both haptics externalized

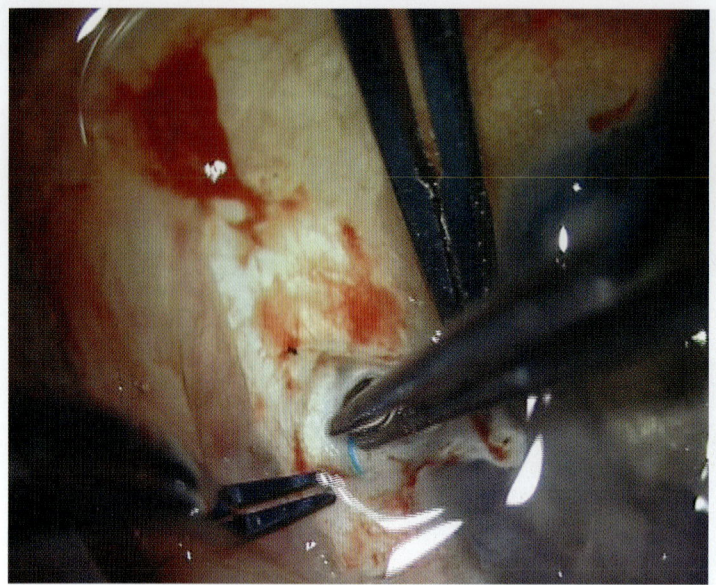

Fig. 10.6 Haptic tucked in Scharioth pocket

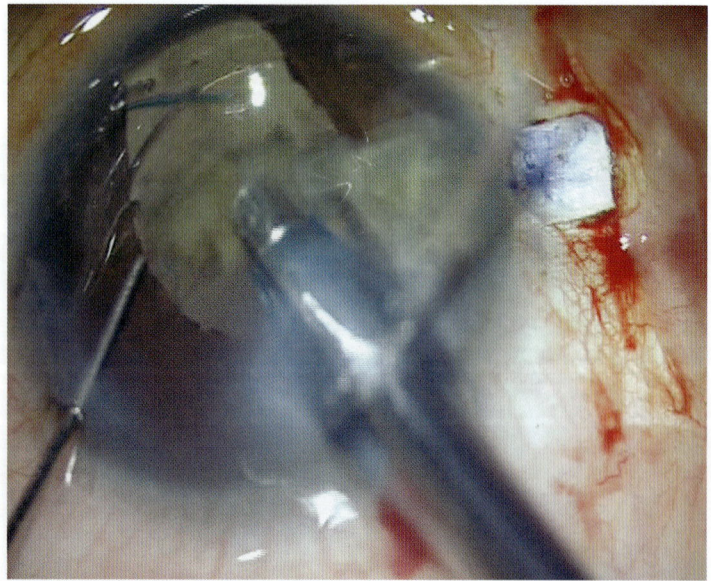

Fig. 10.7 Phaco of the nuclear pieces. Artificial posterior capsule created by the IOL

Glued Intraocular Lens Scaffold

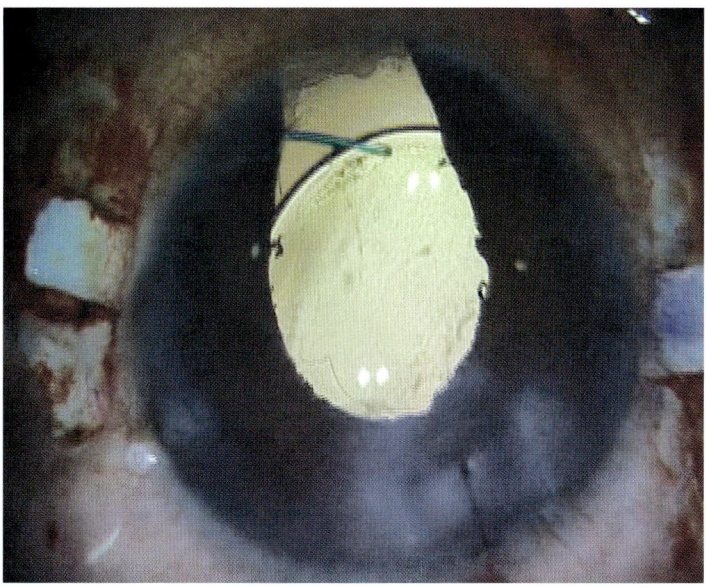

Fig. 10.8 Nucleus emulsified. Note the IOL scaffold and the glued IOL procedure combined prevent the nucleus from falling down. Nucleus totally emulsified

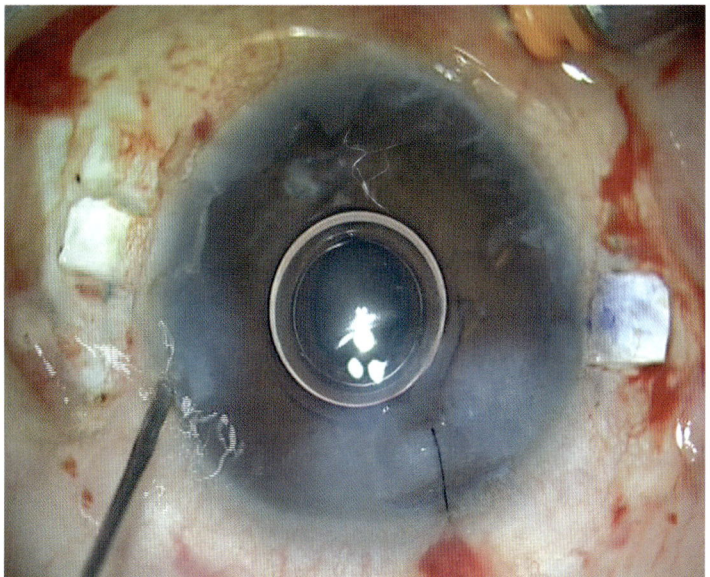

Fig. 10.9 Fibrin glue application to seal the scleral flaps

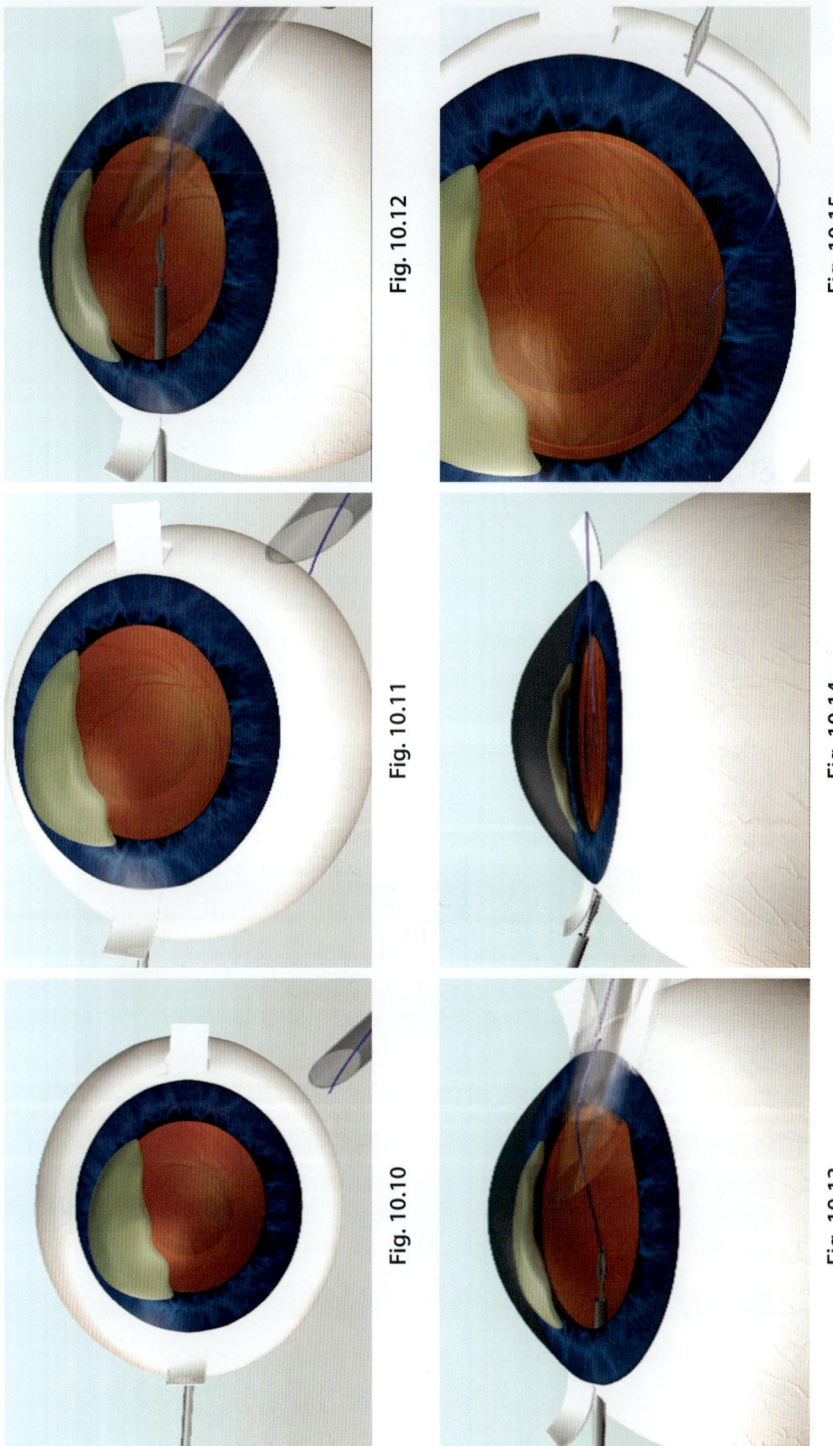

Fig. 10.10

Fig. 10.11

Fig. 10.12

Fig. 10.13

Fig. 10.14

Fig. 10.15

Glued Intraocular Lens Scaffold

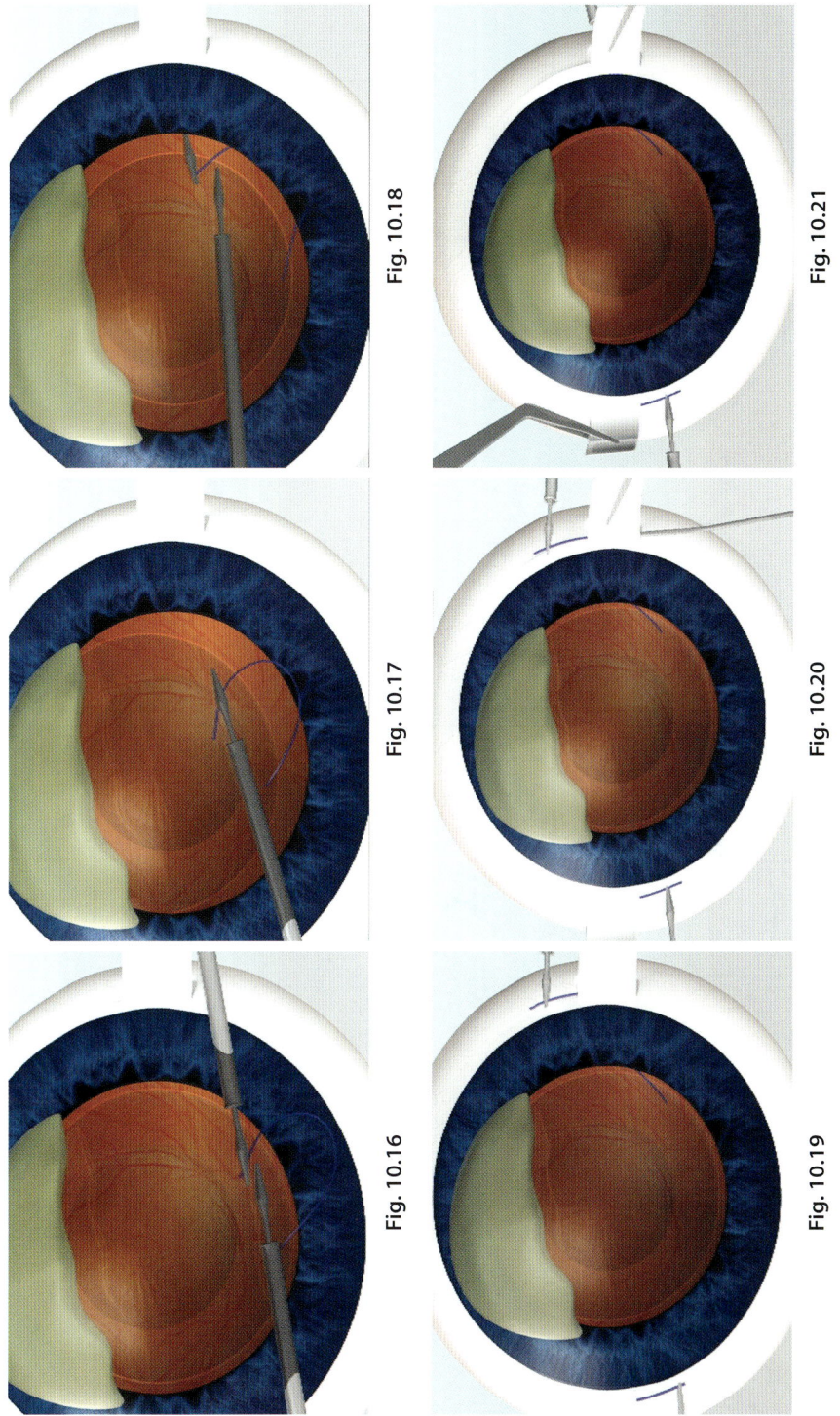

Fig. 10.16

Fig. 10.17

Fig. 10.18

Fig. 10.19

Fig. 10.20

Fig. 10.21

Management of PHACO Complications: Newer Techniques

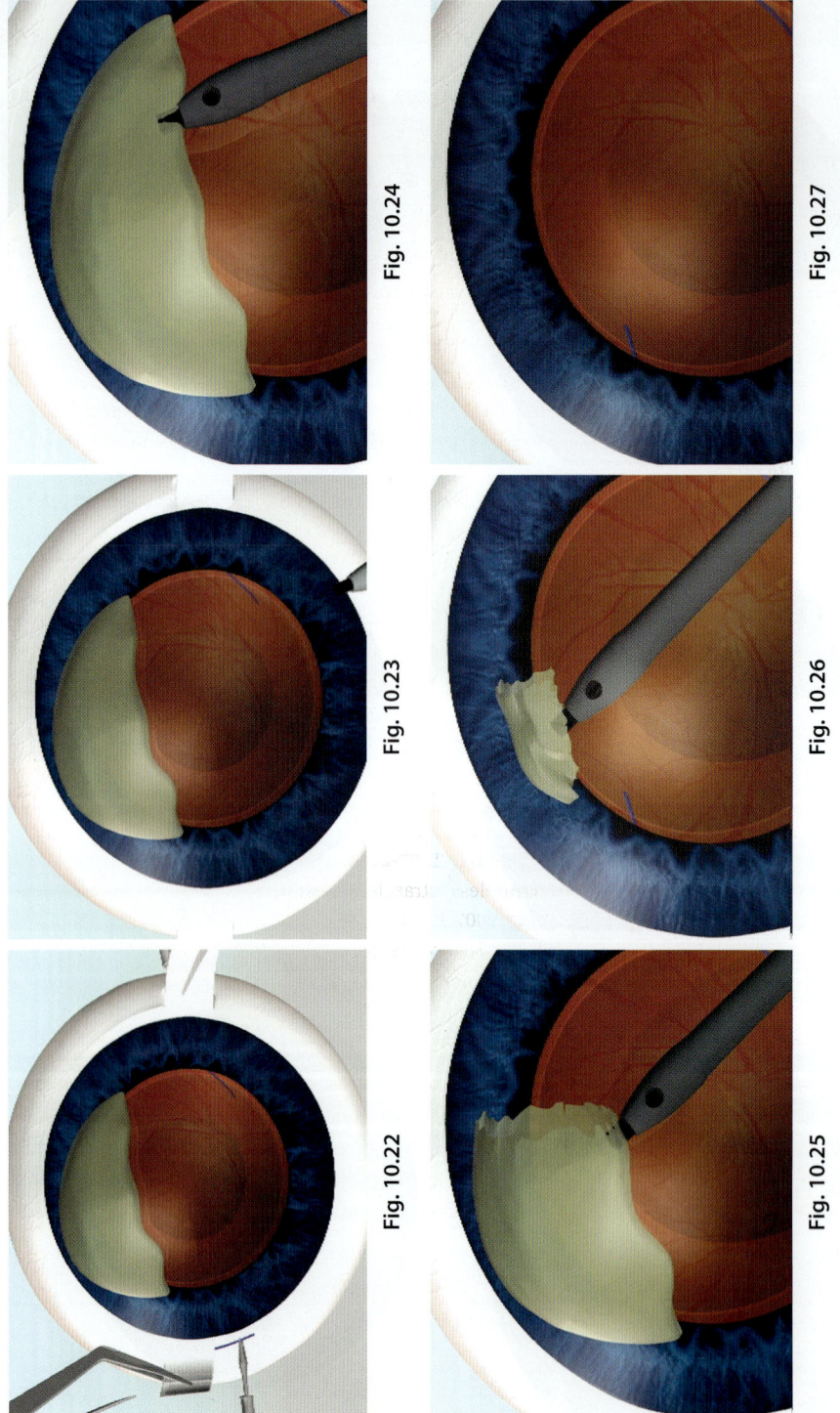

Fig. 10.22 Fig. 10.23 Fig. 10.24

Fig. 10.25 Fig. 10.26 Fig. 10.27

Figs 10.10 to 10.27 Illustrations showing the glued IOL scaffold techniuqe

DIFFICULTIES

The biggest problem encountered during the procedure (Figs 10.10 to 10.27) is the visualization of haptics in cases of large nuclear fragments. Another problem is to be careful of endothelial damage as phacoemulsification procedure is performed in the anterior chamber. Profuse use of viscoelastic is advocated to prevent endothelial damage.

Combining the glued IOL and the IOL scaffold techniques, one can create an artificial posterior capsule in certain select cases of capsular deficiency where the iris is deficient or the pupil is too large to support an IOL.

REFERENCES

1. Agarwal A, Kumar DA, Jacob S, et al. Fibrin glue–assisted sutureless posterior chamber intraocular lens implantation in eyes with deficient posterior capsules. J Cataract Refract Surg. 2008;34:1433-8.
2. Prakash G, Kumar DA, Jacob S, et al. Anterior segment optical coherence tomography-aided diagnosis and primary posterior chamber intraocular lens implantation with fibrin glue in traumatic phacocele with scleral perforation. J Cataract Refract Surg. 2009;35:782-4.
3. Prakash G, Jacob S, Kumar DA, et al. Femtosecond assisted keratoplasty with fibrin glue–assisted sutureless posterior chamber lens implantation: a new triple procedure. J Cataract Refract Surg. In press (manuscript no 08-919).
4. Agarwal A, Kumar DA, Prakash G, et al. Fibrin glue–assisted sutureless posterior chamber intraocular lens implantation in eyes with deficient posterior capsules [Reply to letter]. J Cataract Refract Surg. 2009;35:795-6.
5. Nair V, Kumar DA, Prakash G, et al. Bilateral spontaneous in-the-bag anterior subluxation of PCIOL managed with glued IOL technique: A case report, Eye Contact Lens 2009. In Press (manuscript no ECL-07-281).
6. Gabor SGB, Pavilidis MM. Sutureless intrascleral posterior chamber intraocular lens fixation. J Cataract Refract Surg. 2007;33:1851–4.
7. Kumar DA, Agarwal A, et al. IOL Scaffold technique for posterior capsular rupture. J Refract Surg. 2012;28(5):314-5.

SECTION III

Miscellaneous

CHAPTER 11

Intraocular Lens Scaffold for Intraocular Lens Exchange

Roger Steinert, Brian Little, Priya Narang, Amar Agarwal

INTRODUCTION

Intraocular lens (IOL) exchange after an uneventful cataract surgery calls for a lot of disappointment, frustration and at times a challenge. IOL exchange can be challenging when a portion of the IOL is incarcerated by synechias or when a haptic is imbedded in the angle. Intraocular manipulation of the IOL may result in iris trauma that ranges from mild bleeding to iridodialysis. Refractive surprise is a common indication for IOL exchange. Inaccurate axial length measurement, inaccurate keratometry, wrong eye selection, incorrect IOL packaging can lead to unintended refractive outcome.

Studies have depicted intraoperative complications such as zonular dialysis, posterior capsule rupture (PCR), and iridodialysis in approximately 30 percent of cases,[1-3] reflecting the technical difficulty of IOL exchange procedure. In some cases, an Nd-YAG laser capsulotomy may have been performed, further complicating an IOL exchange.

Various techniques have been devised to decrease the incidence of intraoperative complications in IOL exchange such as removing the optic only, leaving the firmly adhered haptics in the bag.[4] Methods for removing a foldable IOL through a small incision include transecting it with a cutting instrument or refolding the IOL in the anterior chamber and removing it intact with the folding instrument.[5,6,7] However, development of a PCR intraoperatively has been reported when the optic is being divided for removal through a small incision.[4]

Intraocular lens scaffold[8,9] has been described as a technique in cases of PCR wherein the IOL is inserted below the nonemulsified nuclear fragments; the IOL acts as a barrier or scaffold, creating an artificial posterior capsule and preventing the slippage of any nuclear material in the posterior chamber, facilitating safe emulsification in the anterior chamber. A surgical technique that can solve the issue of PCR creation during the process of optic dissection with scissors and/or prevent vitreous prolapse when the posterior capsule is already open prior to the IOL exchange is described. In this technique too, after the offending IOL is elevated into the anterior chamber from the bag, a corrective IOL is injected in the bag; followed by removal of the original IOL.

SURGICAL TECHNIQUE

Adequate pupil dilation is ensured before the surgery and a peribulbar block is administered. A previously created corneal incision is opened if the prior surgery is recent; otherwise a fresh incision in a different location is created. The anterior chamber is filled with an ophthalmic viscosurgical device (OVD) and it is also injected beneath the IOL optic; the capsular bag is safely dissected and separated from the IOL surface using standard techniques. Once some protection of the posterior capsule is obtained, the hook and dialers are used to gently lift the IOL and manipulate the IOL out of the bag (Fig. 11.1). The IOL is slightly pushed to the opposite side so that the haptics can be easily removed out of the bag. In cases where the haptic end cannot be freed from the capsule equator, the haptic is cut as far as possible in the periphery utilizing coaxial action microscissors. A corrective IOL is loaded and injected beneath the previous IOL and dialed into the bag (Fig. 11.2). This new IOL acts as a scaffold when the offending IOL is cut, preventing damage to the posterior capsule, or, in cases where the posterior capsule is already open, acting as a barrier/scaffold to vitreous prolapse. The offending IOL is cut with the help of IOL cutting scissors into two pieces which are then explanted sequentially (Figs 11.3 to 11.5). Ophthalmic viscosurgical device is aspirated and/or irrigated from the eye and the corneal incision is sealed by hydrating the corneal stroma or utilizing a suture as needed.

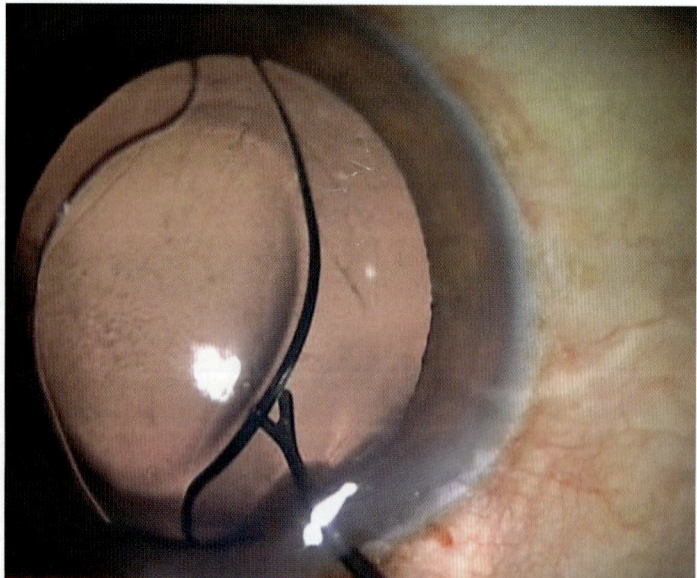

Fig. 11.1 The offending intraocular lens (IOL) is lifted from the bag after adequate injection of viscoelastic behind the IOL offering an adequate protection to the capsular bag

Intraocular Lens Scaffold for Intraocular Lens Exchange

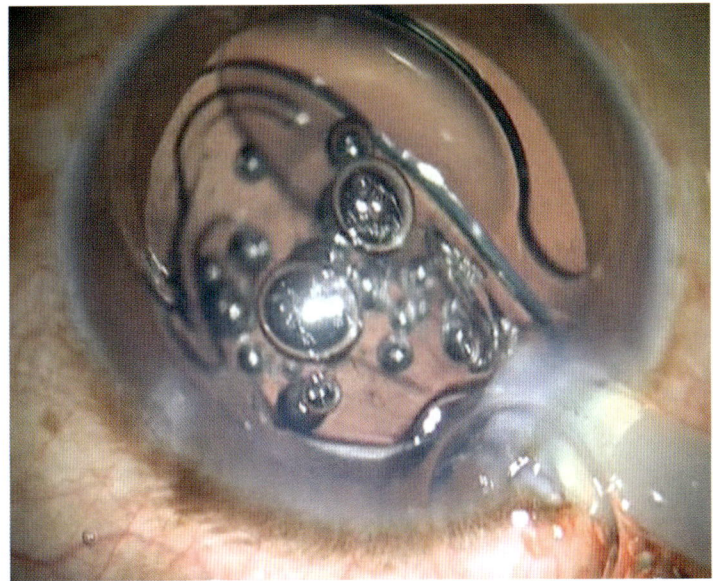

Fig. 11.2 A fresh corrective IOL is injected behind the levitated offending IOL

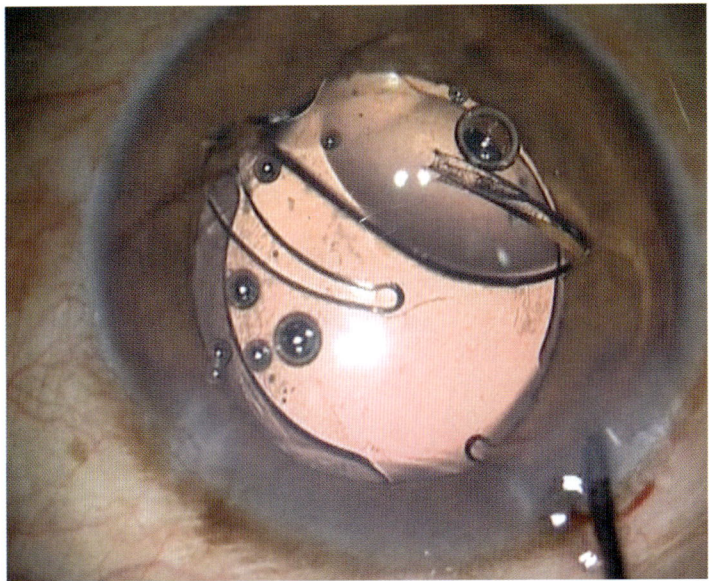

Fig. 11.3 The IOL is being cut with scissors

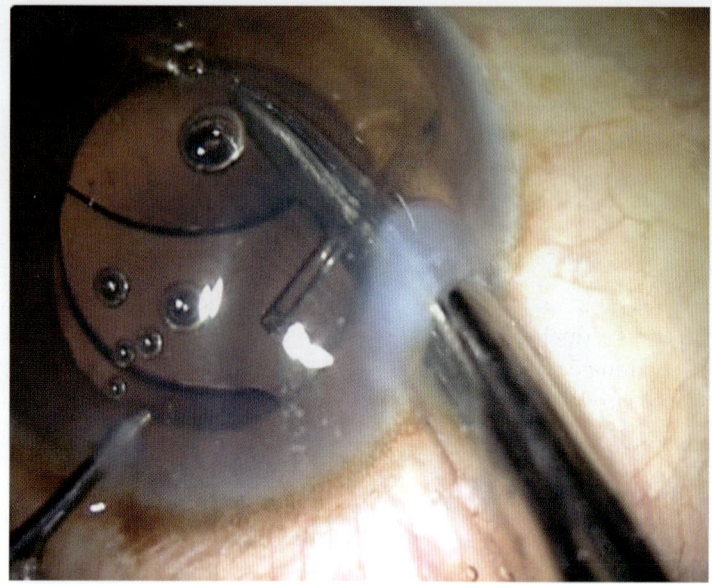

Fig. 11.4 The IOL is rotated 180 degree and the remaining half of the optic is also cut, dividing the optic into two pieces

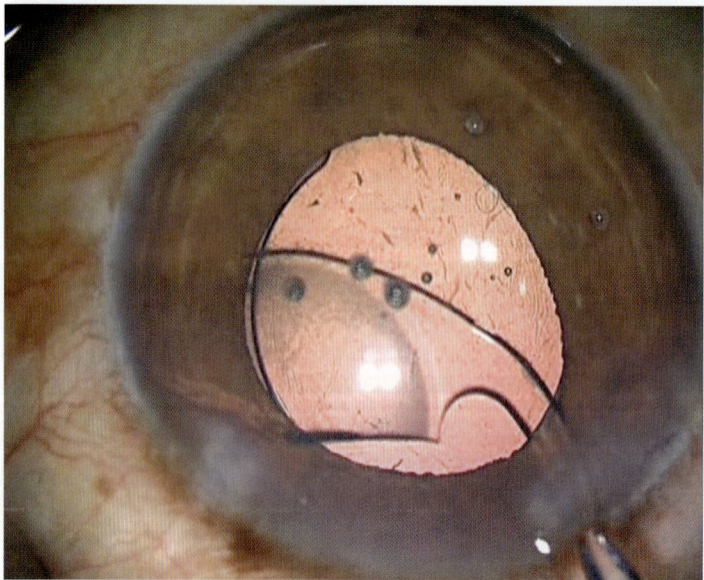

Fig. 11.5 The cut IOL is sequentially explanted

DISCUSSION

This technique involves the presence of 2 IOLs in the eye; the offending IOL being manipulated out of the capsular bag into the anterior chamber followed by insertion of a corrective IOL into the bag. This technique does not require specially designed instruments. The offending levitated IOL into the anterior chamber is transected with the IOL cutting scissors; meanwhile the corrective IOL acts as a scaffold for the posterior capsule. During optic transection, the stability of IOL optic is a major concern to prevent the optic slippage to avoid inadvertent damage to the ocular tissues including the posterior capsule. This technique offers a dual advantage of continuous distention of the bag with IOL thereby preventing damage to the posterior capsule due to barrier effect, acting as a barrier to vitreous prolapse in cases of already open posterior capsule, and preventing any slippage of the optic during the process of transection of the IOL being removed.

Meticulous separation of the IOL from the capsular bag with viscoelastic material followed by its prolapse into the anterior chamber and insertion of a fresh IOL into the bag is a key to the success of the procedure. Although the pieces with attached haptics may be slightly larger, their flexibility allows them to be withdrawn easily, with virtually no deformation as they pass through the wound.

REFERENCES

1. Yu AKF, Ng ASY. Complications and clinical outcomes of intraocular lens exchange in patients with calcified hydrogel lenses. J Cataract Refract Surg. 2002;28:1217-22.
2. Gashau AG, Anand A, Chawdhary S. Hydrophilic acrylic intraocular lens exchange: five-year experience. J Cataract Refract Surg. 2006;32:1340-4.
3. Voros GM, Strong NP. Exchange technique for opacified hydrophilic acrylic intraocular lenses. Eur J Ophthalmol. 2005;15:465-7.
4. Lee SJ, Sun HJ, Choi KS, Park HS. Intraocular lens exchange with removal of the optic only. JCRS, 2009;35:514-8.
5. Koch H-R. Lens bisector for silicone intraocular lens removal. J Cataract Refract Surg. 1996;22:1379-80.
6. Koo EY, Lindsey PS, Soukiasian SH. Bisecting a foldable acrylic intraocular lens for explantation. J Cataract Refract Surg. 1996;22:1381-2.
7. Neuhann TH. Intraocular folding of an acrylic lens for explantation through a small incision cataract wound. J Cataract Refract Surg. 1996;22:1383-6.
8. Kumar DA, Agarwal A, Prakash G, Jacob S, Agarwal A, Sivagnanam S. IOL scaffold technique for posterior capsule rupture.[letter] J Refract Surg. 2012;28:314-5.
9. Narang P, Agarwal A, Kumar DA, Jacob S, Agarwal A, Agarwal A. Clinical outcomes of intraocular lens scaffold surgery. A one-year study. Ophthalmology. 2013;120:2442-8.

CHAPTER **12**

Pre-Descemet's Endothelial Keratoplasty

Harminder Dua, Priya Narang, Amar Agarwal

Endothelial keratoplasty (EK) has evolved at a brisk pace and the volume of data accumulated over the past 10 years has demonstrated that all the posterior lamellar techniques of endothelial replacement yield far superior visual, topographic, and tectonic results compared with penetrating keratoplasty.[1] A novel method of EK in which the endothelium and Descemet's membrane (DM) along with the Pre-Descemet's layer (Dua's layer-PDL) is transplanted is described hereby and it has been termed as pre-Descemet's endothelial keratoplasty (PDEK). Early evidence to support the existence of a distinct pre-Descemet's layer of tissue was presented by Dua et al[2] in 2007 and followed by a detailed paper wherein evidence is presented to further support the presence of the distinct PDL. In PDEK procedure, this layer is included with the endothelium—DM complex thereby providing additional support to the graft. Presence of this layer with its characteristics of relative rigidity and toughness allows easy intraoperative handling and insertion of the tissue as it does not tend to scroll as much as the DM alone. The most popular in 'DM barring' techniques is the big bubble (BB) method where the BB forms a cleavage plane, leaving the DM bare for the dissection in lamellar keratoplasties. This entails the creation of Type 2 big bubble where the bubble forms between the PDL and the DM. In PDEK procedure, Type 1 big bubble[2] is formed which typically lies between the PDL and the residual corneal stroma; thereby creating a dome of PDL-DM-endothelial complex above the air bubble.

SURGICAL TECHNIQUE

Donor Graft Preparation

A graft with a 2 mm corneoscleral rim all around the cornea is dissected from the whole globe. With the endothelial side up, a 30 G needle attached to a 2 mL air-filled syringe is introduced with a bevel up position from the corneoscleral rim into the mid-periphery of the cornea followed by injection of air. A 7 to 8.5 mm Type 1 bubble is created which spreads from the center to periphery; with a distinct rim all around (Fig. 12.1A). Trephination of the donor graft is done along

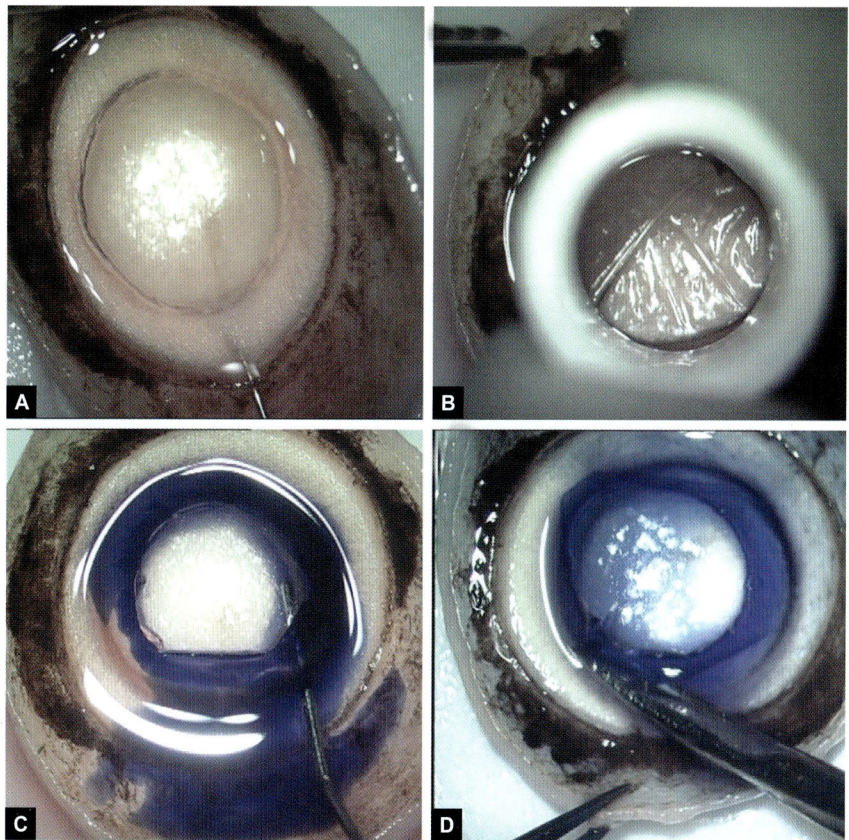

Figs 12.1A to D (A) Type 1 bubble created by injecting air from a 30 gauge needle introduced from the corneoscleral rim; (B) Trephination has done of the donor graft; (C) Trypan blue injected into the air bubble; (D) Donor graft cut with corneoscleral scissors along the edges of the bubble

the margin of the big bubble (Fig. 12.1B). The bubble wall is penetrated at the extreme periphery and trypan blue is injected into the bubble to stain the graft (Fig. 12.1C), which is then cut all around the trephine mark with a pair of corneoscleral scissors (Fig. 12.1D). The graft is then placed in the storage medium and is loaded on to an injector of a foldable intraocular lens when ready for insertion.

Recipient Bed Preparation

The surgery is performed after administering peribulbar anesthesia (10 mL 2% xylocaine and 0.75% L-bupivacaine combined with 100 IU hyaluronidase). A trephine mark is made on the recipient cornea respective to the diameter of DM to be scored on the endothelial side (Figs 12.2A and B). A 2.8 mm corneal tunnel incision is made entering the anterior chamber just at the mark. Air is injected

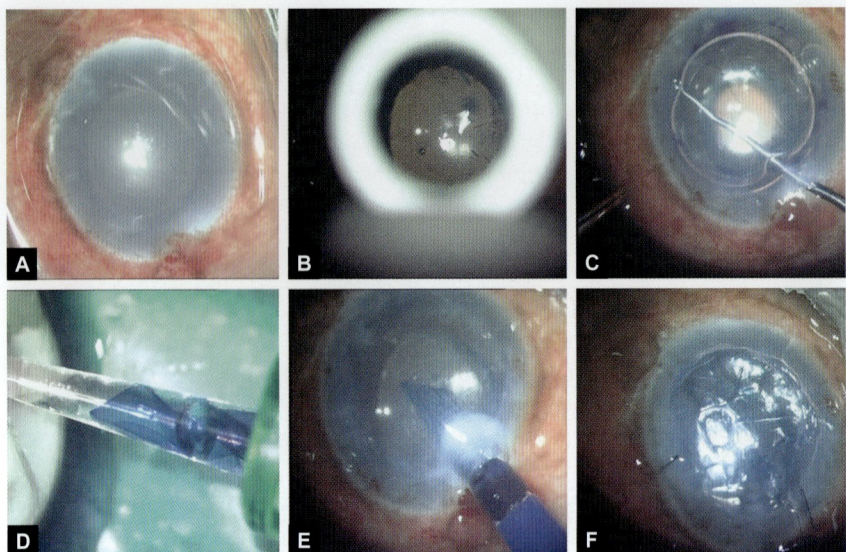

Figs 12.2A to F (A) The edematous recipient cornea; (B) Trephination of the recipient cornea; (C) Descemetorhexis has done along the margin of trephine mark; (D) Trypan blue stained graft is loaded on to the injector; (E) The loaded graft being injected into the anterior chamber (AC); (F) Air injected beneath the graft so as to fill the AC. Corneal suture taken to ensure AC stability

into the anterior chamber and with a reverse Sinskey hook, a circular portion of DM is stripped from the posterior stroma, so that descemetorhexis is created (Fig. 12.2C), and the portion of stripped DM is removed from the eye. Once an adequate edge is lifted, a nontoothed forceps is used to gently grab the Descemet's membrane at its very edge and the graft is separated from the underlying stroma in a capsulorhexis-like circumferential manner.

Graft Injection

The donor pre-Descemet's roll which is previously stained with a 0.06 percent trypan blue solution is loaded into the foldable injector and is inserted into the anterior chamber (Figs 12.2D and E) where it is gently spread out. This donor disk is then uncoiled using fluidics and the surgeon must avoid for the most part any direct instrument contact to the donor endothelium. Proper orientation is essential prior to attaching the donor pre-Descemet's roll to the exposed recipient bare corneal stroma. The graft orientation is then checked and it is unfolded gently using a small air-bubble as described by Melles. Once unfolded, an adequately tight air bubble is injected under the graft to float it up against the stroma.

An air bubble is injected underneath the donor DM to lift the DM onto the recipient posterior stroma. The anterior chamber is filled with air (Fig. 12.2F). Eye speculum is finally removed and AC is examined for air position. The patient is advised to lie in a strictly supine position for next 3 hours.

DISCUSSION

Pre-Descemet's endothelial keratoplasty (PDEK) entails the inclusion of the PDL in the donor graft; thereby providing the benefits of Descemet's membrane endothelial keratoplasty (DMEK) like speedy visual recovery and overcoming the disadvantages posed by DMEK. Pre-Descemet's endothelial keratoplasty (PDEK) takes ultra thin-Descemet's stripping endothelial keratoplasty (UT-DSEK) to a 'thinner level' whilst retaining its advantages but not requiring sophisticated instrumentation and keratome. The spectral domain optical coherence tomography (SD-OCT) *in vivo* analysis of PDEK grafts showed mean graft thickness after 1 month to be 28±5.6 microns which is larger than the conventional DMEK graft and lesser than the ultrathin Descemet's stripping automated endothelial keratoplasty (DSAEK) graft. In PDEK, the additional layer thickness with endothelium-DM complex is lesser than the overall thickness of the DSEK or ultrathin DSAEK graft. This is compatible with a faster visual recovery. A comparison of the preoperative and postoperative clinical slit lamp pictures of the eye along with OCT images show a clear graft on the first postoperative day (Figs 12.3A to C). Some aspects of the different endothelial keratoplasty techniques are demonstrated in Table 12.1.

The major shortcoming of this technique is the size of graft which is around 8 mm; allowing a slightly limited access to the donor endothelium complex as compared to other techniques. This may however be compensated by reduced cell loss related to manipulation of tissue. Importantly, PDEK will allow use of younger donor eyes, less than 50 years, which are not suitable for harvesting

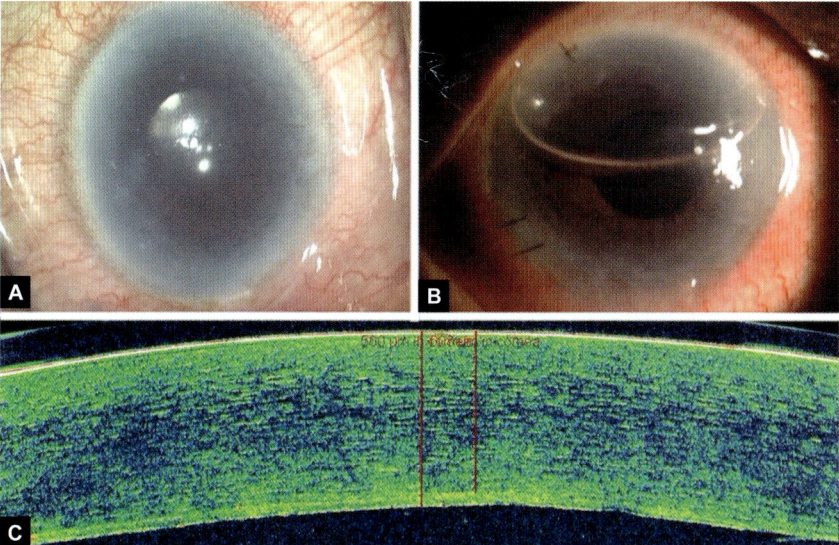

Figs 12.3A to C Preoperative and postoperative picture of patient with optical coherence tomography (OCT) image

TABLE 12.1 Comparison of the different endothelial keratoplasty techniques

	DSEK	DMEK	PDEK
Surgical layers	Stroma + Dm + Endo	Dm + Endo	Pre-Descemet's + Dm + Endo
Technical difficulty	Easy	Difficult	Moderate
Type of procedure	Tissue additive	Tissue neutral	Minimal tissue additive
Artificial anterior chamber	Required	NR	NR
Microkeratome	Required (DSAEK)	NR	NR
Induced hyperopia	Yes	No	No
Corneal thickness	Increased	Normal	Minimal
Intrastromal interface	Yes	No	Minimal
Cost	Costly	Cost effective	Cost effective
Eye bank prepared donor tissue	Available	No	Can be made available
Graft unrolling	Easy	Difficult	Moderate
Tissue handling	Good	Difficult	Good
Visual recovery	Slow	Fast	Fast

Abbreviations:
Dm — Descemet's membrane
Endo — Endothelium
DSAEK — Descemet's stripping automated endothelial keratoplasty
NR — Not required

DMEK tissue. Pre-Descemet's endothelial keratoplasty (PDEK) thus enables the higher cell counts associated with younger donors to be exploited to the patient's advantage. Moreover, endothelial cells are capable of proliferation and acquire morphological adaptations to compensate for the peripheral cornea. Another drawback can be the occasional creation of Type 2 bubble instead of Type 1; necessitating the conversion of PDEK to DMEK in order to prevent the wastage of donor tissue.

Long term studies evaluating different parameters such as endothelial cell loss over time, interface haze, detachment rates and final visual acuity including higher order aberrations and contrast sensitivity are required to establish a place for PDEK in corneal transplantation surgery.

REFERENCES

1. Terry MA. Endothelial Keratoplasty: Why Aren't We All Doing Descemet's Membrane Endothelial Keratoplasty? Cornea. 2012;31(5)469:71.
2. Dua HS, Faraj LA, Said DG, Gray T, Lowe J. Human Corneal Anatomy Redefined: A Novel Pre-Descemet's Layer (Dua's Layer). Ophthalmology. 2013;120(9):1778-85.

CHAPTER **13**

Negative Dysphotopsia

Samuel Masket, Nicole R Fram

Negative dysphotopsia (ND) represents an undesired optical phenomenon following cataract surgery. It is classically described as a dark temporal shadow. Conversely, positive dysphotopsia (PD) is characterized by light streaks, star bursts or glare. Both photopsias interfere significantly with quality of vision and perceived success of surgery. The dysphotopsias can result in unrelenting patient dissatisfaction after otherwise uncomplicated cataract surgery. Given that ND and PD differ in etiology and management, techniques for treatment should be considered separately. However, both conditions may exist simultaneously.

NEGATIVE DYSPHOTOPSIA

Davison originally described ND in 2000 as complaints of a dark temporal shadow, similar to 'horse blinders.'[1] What is most frustrating to the surgeon and patient alike is that ND is mainly reported in cases where the PCIOL of any design, is well centered within the confines of the capsular bag.

Diagnostic tests to rule out concomitant ocular pathology including visual field testing and a through dilated fundus retinal examination are needed prior to attributing symptoms to persistent ND. Unfortunately, medical treatment has not been shown to be useful in treating ND. Initial reports implicated temporal corneal incisions as a causative factor in ND,[2] however, ND has been reported with superior incisions.[3] There does, however, appear to be a difference between transient ND and permanent ND which may be related to surgical incision and/or opacification of the lens capsule.[2,4] Previous publications have implicated posterior chamber depth, pupil size, index of refraction, lens material and edge design as causative factors in ND.[4] Vamosi et al concluded that in-the-bag IOL exchange alone did not improve symptoms of ND and posterior chamber depth as examined by UBM was not a significant factor in incidence of ND.[5] However, when iris/optic distance was collapsed with a sulcus placement of IOL during exchange then symptoms of ND were improved. Although the etiology of ND is likely multifactorial, we do know that it can occur with any lens material, is persistent despite collapse of the posterior chamber with an 'in-the-bag' IOL and does not typically improve with in-the bag-IOL exchange. This constellation of findings implicates the anterior capsule/IOL interaction as a possible factor in the etiology of ND.[6]

Surgical methods to address ND includes secondary 'Piggyback' IOL, reverse optic capture (ROC) and/or sulcus placement of a secondary PCIOL have been devised and proven useful in reducing visual symptoms of ND. Although ND rarely induces visual disability sufficient to require an operative approach, some patients are very disturbed and can be very vocal in their complaints. To our understanding, ND has never been reported with sulcus placed PCIOLs or ACIOLs. In our investigation, we found that ND occurs only with 'in-the-bag' PCIOLs with overlap of the anterior capsulorhexis onto the anterior surface of the PCIOL.[6] We do not believe that the corneal incision plays a role in persistent ND.[3]

Given the above, and in keeping with our studies, two surgical strategies have emerged as beneficial—reverse optic capture (ROC) and placement of a secondary 'Piggyback' IOL. Failed surgical strategies include within the bag IOL exchange wherein the original implant is removed and another of different material, shape or edge design is replaced within the capsule bag. This is in keeping with the work of Vamosi, et al.[5]

One successful surgical method, reverse optic capture (ROC), may be employed in a secondary surgery for symptomatic patients, or as a primary prophylactic strategy. In cases of the latter, the method has been applied to the second eye of patients who were significantly symptomatic following routine uncomplicated surgery in their first eye. It should be noted, however, that ND symptoms are not necessarily bilateral.

Secondary ROC, performed for symptomatic patients, may be applied if the anterior capsulotomy is not too small or too thick or rigid from postoperative fibrosis. At surgery, the anterior capsule is freed from the underlying optic by gentle blunt and viscodissection (Fig. 13.1). Next, the nasal anterior capsule edge is retracted with one Sinskey hook (or similar device) while the optic edge is elevated and the capsule edge allowed to slip under the optic (Fig. 13.2). This maneuver is repeated 180 degrees away temporally, leaving the haptics undisturbed in the bag (Figs 13.3 to 13.5). Primary or prophylactic ROC is performed at the time of initial cataract surgery for the symptomatic patient's second eye. It should be recognized that surgical success in achieving primary or secondary ROC is highly dependent on a properly sized and centered anterior capsulorhexis. There seems to be little optical consequence of ROC, as the haptics remain in the bag; theoretically, however a modest myopic shift would be induced, varying directly with the power of the IOL.

The other surgical method that has proven successful for patients with symptomatic ND is a 'Piggyback' IOL, as first reported by Ernest.[7] In this method, a second IOL is implanted in the ciliary sulcus atop the IOL/capsule bag complex. It appears that covering the primary optic/capsule junction reduces ND symptoms,

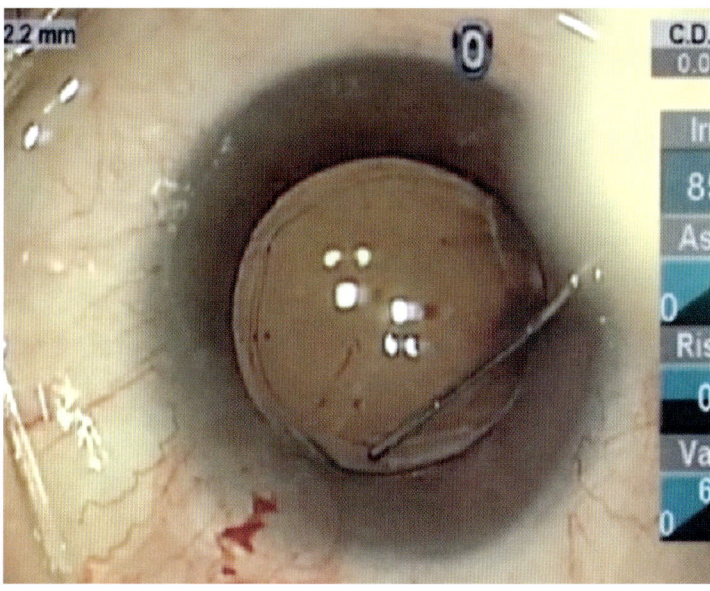

Fig. 13.1 A Sinskey hook is fed underneath the anterior capsule following viscodissection in an attempt to free the optic from the capsule

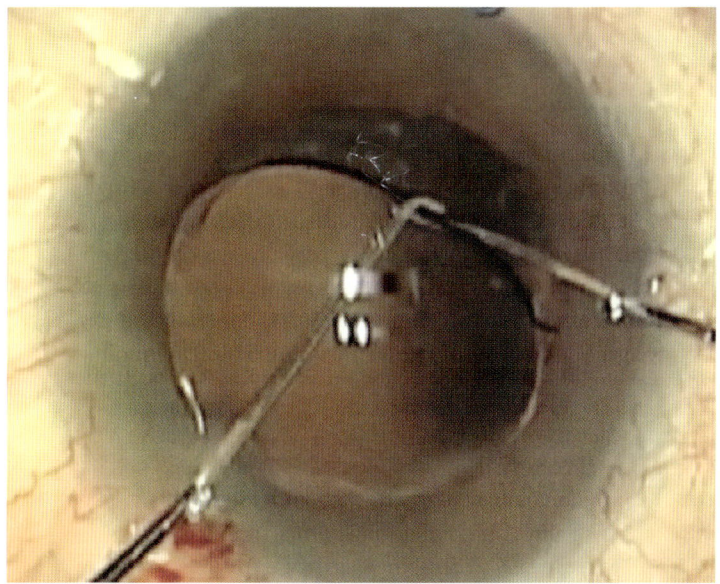

Fig. 13.2 The Sinskey hook and blunt spatula are used to elevate the optic edge over the capsule

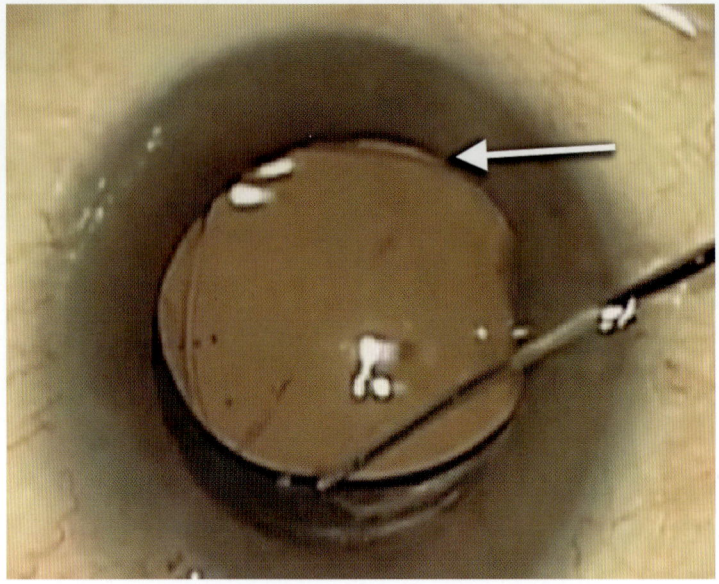

Fig. 13.3 Once the nasal edge has been captured (see arrow), the opposite, temporal edge of the optic is elevated over the anterior capsule edge

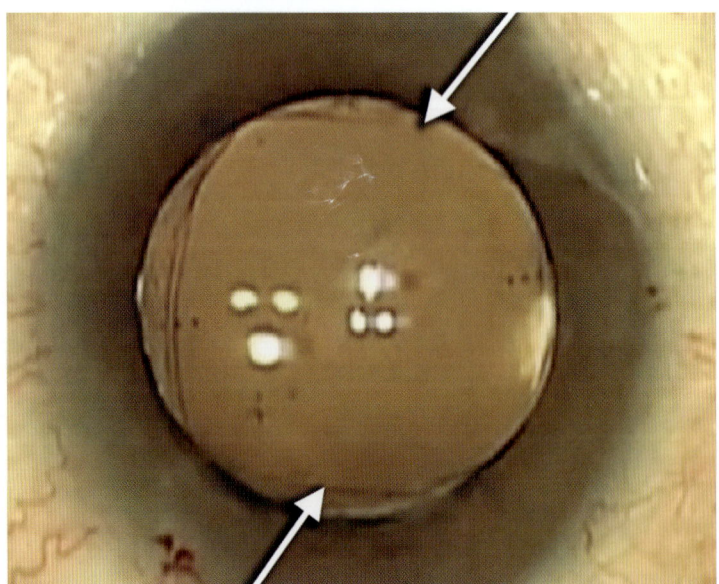

Fig. 13.4 Optic capture has been completed. The nasal and temporal edges of the implant are anterior to the anterior capsule (see arrows), whereas the haptics remain fully within the capsular bag

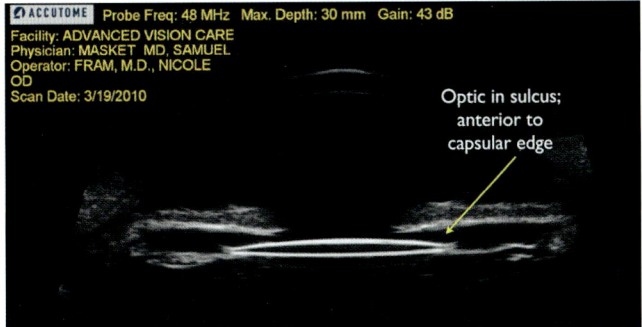

Fig. 13.5 Ultrasound biomicroscopy (UBM) demonstrating reverse optic capture with the optic edge anterior to the capsular edge

although the original concept was that a 'Piggyback' lens was effective because it collapsed the posterior chamber by reducing the distance between the posterior iris and the anterior surface of the IOL. However, our studies have determined that the depth of the posterior chamber is unrelated to ND symptoms.[5, 6] We prefer use of a 3-piece silicone IOL. Regarding ametropia, for hyperopic errors multiply the spectacle error by 1.5 to determine IOL power, while for myopic errors multiply by 1.2. So, as an example, in the case of a 2 D hyperope, implant a + 3.0 D IOL in the ciliary sulcus.

Recent publications have reported improvement of ND symptoms with Nd:YAG capsulectomy of the nasal anterior capsule.[8,9] This treatment, however, may limit future management strategies such as reverse optic capture in the event that the capsulectomy intervention is unsuccessful.

POSITIVE DYSPHOTOPSIA

Positive dysphotopsia (PD) is reported by patients as light streaks, halos, star bursts, etc. It may be induced by internal reflections from either the optic edge or optic surfaces.[10] Therefore, PD appears to be related directly to IOL material, optic size index of refraction, radius of curvature, surface reflectivity, and edge design. Typically, PD is associated with thick square edge design, high index of refraction, low radius of curvature and high surface reflectivity.[11,12] Unlike ND, patients may perceive benefit from use of miotic agents, particularly under dim light conditions. Medical management of PD includes brimonidine tartrate 0.15 percent can be tried initially; also useful is a dilute solution of pilocarpine, typically 0.5 percent. While topical miotics may be helpful, they are associated with the potential for allergies and side effects.

Should miotic therapy prove unsuccessful, and the symptoms mandate further treatment, IOL exchange may be highly successful. In this situation, opt for a lens with a low index of refraction, large optic diameter, and a thin round edge design.

Patients with either ND or PD require careful and concerned attention to their symptoms, a meaningful discussion of the suspected etiology, and should be presented with a supportive plan for assistance.

REFERENCES

1. Davison JA. Positive and negative dysphotopsia in patients with acrylic intraocular lenses. J Cataract Refract Surg. 2000;26:1346-55.
2. Osher RH. Negative dysphotopsia: long-term study and possible explanation for transient symptoms. J Cataract Refract Surg. 2008;34(10):1699-707. doi: 10.1016/j.jcrs.2008.06.026.
3. Cooke DL. Negative dysphotopsia after temporal corneal incisions. J Cataract Refract Surg. 2010;36:671-2.
4. Holladay JT, Zhao H, Reisin CR. Negative dysphotopsia: the enigmatic penumbra. J Cataract Refract Surg. 2012;38:1251-65.
5. Vamosi P, Csakany B, Nemeth K. Intraocular lens exchange in patients with negative dysphotopsia symptoms. J Cataract Refract Surg. 2010;36:418-24.
6. Masket S, Fram NR. Pseudophakic Negative Dysphotopsia: Surgical Management and New Theory of Etiology. J Cataract Refract Surg. 2011;37(7):1199-207.
7. Ernest PH. Severe photic phenomenon. J Cataract Refract Surg. 2006;32:685-6.
8. Cooke DL, Kasko S, Platt LO. Resolution of negative dysphotopsia after laser anterior capsulotomy. J Cataract Refract Surg. 2013;39:1107-9.
9. Folden DV. Neodymium:YAG laser anterior capsulectomy: Surgical option in the management of negative dysphotopsia. J Cataract Refract Surg. 2013;39:1110-5.
10. Holladay JT, Lang A, Portney V. Analysis of edge glare phenomena in intraocular lens edge designs. J Cataract Refract Surg. 1999;25:748-52.
11. Masket S. Truncated edge design, dysphotopsia, and inhibition of posterior capsule opacification. J Cataract Refract Surg. 2000;26(1):145-7.
12. Masket S, Geraghty E, Crandall AS, et al. Undesired light images associated with ovoid intraocular lenses. J Cataract Refract Surg. 1993;19:690-4.

Index

Page numbers followed by *f* refer to figure

A

Agarwal's modification of Malyugin ring 16, 20*f*, 21*f*
Agarwal-Katena' forceps 16, 17*f*, 19*f*
Ahmed micrograsper 70*f*
Air pump 4
Anterior
    bimanual vitrectomy 14
    chamber maintainer 50
    segment ocular coherence tomography 63*f*
    vented gas forced infusion system 6
    vitrectomy 32*f*
Artificial anterior chamber 114

B

Balanced salt solution 3, 5, 84
Beiko's
    and Steinert's modification 77
    modification 78*f*
Bimanual
    irrigation-aspiration of cortex 90
    pars plana anterior vitrectomy 90
    vitrectomy 14*f*

C

Capsular bag 106*f*, 118*f*
Choice of
    forceps tips 79
    tissue glue 77
Chopstick technique 16
Conjunctival peritomy 47, 48*f*
Continuous infusion 5
Corneal thickness 114
Cystoid macular edema 40

D

Descemet's
    layer 110
    membrane 110, 114
        endothelial keratoplasty 113
        stripping automated endothelial keratoplasty 113, 114
Descemetorhexis 112*f*
Dislocated intraocular lens 39
Dry cortical aspiration 13

E

Edematous recipient cornea 112*f*
Endothelial keratoplasty 110
    techniques 114
Extended rhexis 10, 11

F

FAVIT' technique 30
Fibrin glue 59
    application 97*f*
Foldable intraocular lens injectors 52

G

Gas forced infusion 3
Glued
    intraocular lens
        forceps 53*f*, 66*f*, 68*f*

scaffold technique 92, 100*f*
surgery 93*f*
technique 72
intrascleral haptic fixation of intraocular lens 47
posterior chamber intraocular lens 92
Graft injection 112

H

Handshake technique 68*f*, 69
   for foldable glued IOL 67
   for glued IOL 65
Horizontal movement of haptic 61*f*
Hydrodelineation 11*f*
Hypotony 84

I

Infusion with
   anterior chamber maintainer 50
   trocar cannula 49
Internal gas forced infusion 6
Intraocular
   lens 89*f*
      exchange 105
      implantation 16
      scaffold 87, 105
   pressure 6, 7, 10, 90
Intraoperative
   dropped nucleus 31*f*
   posterior capsular rupture 93*f*
Intrascleral haptic tuck 57
Intrastromal interface 114
IOL scaffold technique 89*f*

L

Leading haptic externalization 53, 65
Lowering aspiration 13

M

Macular edema 17
Malyugin ring 16

Management of posterior capsular rupture 12
Microkeratome 114
Microvitreoretinal blade 25

N

Needle-guided intrascleral fixation of posterior chamber intraocular lens for aphakia correction 77
No-anesthesia cataract surgery 6
No-assistant technique 72, 73*f*, 74, 75*f*

O

Ocular coherence tomography 62*f*
Offending intraocular lens 106*f*
Ohta's
   IOL haptic gripping forceps 83*f*
   Y-fixation technique 80*f*
   Y-marker for intrascleral IOL fixation technique 82*f*
Ophthalmic viscosurgical device 25, 106
Optic of intraocular lens 41*f*
Optical coherence tomography 113*f*

P

Pars plicata 25*f*
   anterior vitrectomy 23
   vitrectomy 26*f*
Phaco of nuclear pieces 96*f*
Piggyback' IOL 116
Polymethylmethacrylate 52
Posterior
   capsular
      rent 47
      rupture 10, 13*f*, 16, 23, 87, 92, 105
      tear 14*f*
   capsule 16
   polar cataract 11*f*
   segment vitrectomy 32*f*
Pre-Descemet's endothelial keratoplasty 110, 113
Pseudophacodonesis 62
Pupil snap sign 12

Index

R

Removal of nuclear fragments 13*f*
Retinal detachment 17
Reverse optic capture 116
Role of fibrin glue 59

S

Scharioth
    scleral pocket 57
    tuck and glue 67
Scleral
    flap 48, 51
    pocket 58*f*
    thickness flaps 49*f*
Sclerotomies under flap 51
Sclerotomy 25*f*, 50, 52
Seal scleral flaps 97
Sequelae after posterior capsular rupture 16
Signs of posterior capsular rupture 12
Sinskey hook 116, 117*f*
Sleeveless
    extrusion 41*f*
    phacotip assisted levitation of dropped nucleus 30
Spectral domain optical coherence tomography 113
Stability of intraocular lens haptic 60
Subretinal fluid 39
Surgical technique of Ohta's Y-fixation technique 81*f*

T

Toshihiko Ohta's Y-fixation technique 79
Trailing haptic externalization 55, 65
    in no-assistant technique 76*f*
Trephination of recipient cornea 112*f*
Trocar cannula 25*f*, 50, 93*f*
Type of cataract 10, 11

U

Ultrasound biomicroscopy 119*f*
Ultra-thin-Descemet's stripping endothelial keratoplasty 113
U-shaped hook for intrascleral IOL fixation technique 83*f*
Uveitis-glaucoma-hyphema syndrome 62

V

Vertical glued intraocular lens 77
Viscoat
    Pal' technique 30
    trap 90
Viscoexpression 13
Vitrectomy 40*f*, 51, 52, 55, 94*f*
Vitreolenticular adhesions 32*f*, 40*f*
Vitreous traction 16
Vitritis 18

W

White to white measurement 47

Y

Y-shaped incision 79